Innovating for **Patient Safety** in Medicine

Editors:

Rebecca Lawton and Gerry Armitage

Series Editors:

Judy McKimm and Kirsty Forrest

⑤SAGE | 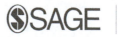 LearningMatters

Learning Matters
An imprint of SAGE Publications Ltd
1 Oliver's Yard
55 City Road
London EC1Y 1SP

SAGE Publications Inc.
2455 Teller Road
Thousand Oaks, California 91320

SAGE Publications India Pvt Ltd
B 1/I 1 Mohan Cooperative Industrial Area
Mathura Road
New Delhi 110 044

SAGE Publications Asia-Pacific Pte Ltd
3 Church Street
#10-04 Samsung Hub
Singapore 049483

Editor: Becky Taylor
Development editor: Richenda Milton-Daws
Production controller: Chris Marke
Project management: Swales & Willis Ltd,
Exeter, Devon
Marketing manager: Tamara Navaratnam
Cover design: Wendy Scott
Typeset by: Swales & Willis Ltd, Exeter, Devon
Printed by: MPG Books Group, Bodmin, Cornwall

First published 2012
Reprinted 2012

Library of Congress Control Number:
2012938956

British Library Cataloguing in Publication data

A catalogue record for this book is available
from the British Library

ISBN 978 0 85725 864 9
ISBN 978 0 85725 765 9 (pbk)

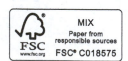

Innovating for Patient Safety in Medicine

Titles in the Series

Health, Behaviour and Society: Clinical Medicine in Context ISBN 9780857254610
Innovating for Patient Safety in Medicine ISBN 9780857257659
Law and Ethics in Medical Practices ISBN 9780857250988
Professional Practice for Foundation Doctors ISBN 9780857252845
Research Skills for Medical Students ISBN 9780857256010
Succeeding in Your Medical Degree ISBN 9780857253972

Contents

Foreword from the Series Editors

Medical education is currently experiencing yet another period of change, typified in the UK with the introduction of the revised *Tomorrow's Doctors* (General Medical Council, 2009) and ongoing work on establishing core curricula for many subject areas. Changes are also occurring at Foundation and postgraduate levels in terms of the introduction of broader non-technical competencies, a wider range of assessments and revalidation requirements. This new series of textbooks has been developed as a direct response to these changes and the impact on all levels of medical education.

Research indicates that effective medical practitioners combine excellent, up-to-date clinical and scientific knowledge with practical skills and the ability to work with patients, families and other professionals with empathy and understanding; they know when to lead and when to follow and they work collaboratively and professionally to improve health outcomes for individuals and communities. In *Tomorrow's Doctors*, the General Medical Council has defined a series of learning outcomes set out under three headings:

1. Doctor as Practitioner;

2. Doctor as Scholar and Scientist;

3. Doctor as Professional.

The books in this series do not cover practical clinical procedures or knowledge about diseases and conditions, but instead cover the range of non-technical professional skills (plus underpinning knowledge) that students and doctors need to know in order to become effective, safe and competent practitioners.

Aimed specifically at medical students (but also of use for junior doctors, teachers and clinicians), each book relates to specific outcomes of *Tomorrow's Doctors* (and, where relevant, the Foundation curriculum), providing both knowledge and help to improve the skills necessary to be successful at the non-clinical aspects of training as a doctor. One of the aims of the series is to set medical practice within the wider social, policy and organisational agendas to help produce future doctors who are socially aware and willing and prepared to engage in broader issues relating to healthcare delivery.

Individual books in the series outline the key theoretical approaches and policy agendas relevant to that subject, and go further by demonstrating through case studies and scenarios how these theories can be used in work settings to achieve best practice. Plenty of activities and self-assessment tools throughout the book will help readers to hone their critical thinking and reflection skills.

Chapters in each of the books follow a standard format. At the beginning a box highlights links to relevant competencies and outcomes from *Tomorrow's Doctors* and other medical curricula, if appropriate. This sets the scene and enables readers to see exactly what will be covered. This is extended by a chapter overview which sets out the key topics and what students should expect to have learnt by the end of the chapter.

There is at least one case study in each chapter which considers how theory can be used in practice from different perspectives. Activities are included which include practical tasks with learning points, critical thinking research tasks and reflective practice/thinking points. Activities can be carried out by readers or with others and are designed to raise awareness, consolidate understanding of theories and ideas and enable students to improve their practice by using models, approaches and ideas. Each activity is followed by a brief discussion on issues raised. At the end of each chapter a chapter summary provides an aide-mémoire of what has been covered.

All chapters are evidence-based in that they set out the theories or evidence that underpins practice. In most chapters, one or more 'What's the evidence?' boxes provide further information about a particular piece of research or a policy agenda through books, articles, websites or policy papers. A list of additional readings is set out under the 'Going further' section, with all references collated at the end of the book.

The series is edited by Professor Judy McKimm and Dr Kirsty Forrest, both of whom are experienced medical educators and writers. Book and chapter authors are drawn from a wide pool of practising clinicians and educators from the UK and internationally.

Author Biographies

Gerry Armitage, Professor, Health Services Research, at the School of Health, University of Bradford and Senior Research Fellow at the Bradford Institute for Health Research. Gerry is also a founder member of the Yorkshire Quality and Safety Research group. Gerry worked as a nurse for over 13 years before moving into nursing education. In the last 10 years he has worked almost entirely in the field of patient safety research and education.

John Bibby, General Practitioner. John has been involved with undergraduate and postgraduate medical education for the past 30 years since being a GP. Over the past 15 years he has been involved in quality improvement in health services nationally and internationally. For the past 10 years he has been involved in patient safety in primary and secondary care and is involved in running the Training and Action on Patient Safety (TAPS) programme.

Ikhlaq Din, Research Fellow, Bradford Institute for Health Research. Ikhlaq has worked as a health researcher for many years. He has particular experience in conducting social and health research with minority ethnic communities as well as engaging with 'marginalised' and excluded communities in Bradford. He has good links with the local population and community organisations in Bradford.

Peter Gardner, Senior Lecturer in Statistics and Human Factors, Institute of Psychological Sciences, University of Leeds. Peter is a human factors psychologist who is keen to apply psychological theory and research to applied issues including the design and implementation of medical devices, new health technology, patient safety and e-health.

Sally Giles, Senior Research Fellow, Bradford Institute for Health Research. Sally is a health services researcher with both qualitative and quantitative research skills and experience. Over the last 10 years she has led and worked on a variety of research projects in the NHS, some of which include research into incident reporting systems, correct site surgery, inpatient falls, shared electronic health records and crisis resolution in mental health.

Angela Grange, Lead Nurse, Clinical Quality & Research/Trust Lead for Innovation, Bradford Teaching Hospitals NHS Foundation Trust. Angela is a qualified children's nurse/general nurse with a background in health services research. She currently leads the development of research capacity and capability building for nurses and midwives, and the strategic development and the implementation of innovations in healthcare in her organisation.

Susan Hrisos, Senior Research Associate, Institute of Health and Society, Newcastle University. Susan is a behavioural scientist who has worked in the field of health services research and implementation science for many years. She has a particular interest in the patient role for the uptake of research findings into clinical practice and for improving the quality and safety of their healthcare.

Vikram Jha, Professor of Medical Education and Head of Undergraduate School of Medicine, University of Liverpool. Vikram is a medical educationalist and consultant obstetrician, with research interests in patient safety, workplace learning and professionalism.

Rebecca Lawton, Professor, Psychology of Healthcare, University of Leeds and Bradford Institute for Health Research. Rebecca is a founder member of the Yorkshire Quality and Safety Research group, one of the leading patient safety research groups in the UK. Her research and teaching career have focused on the application of psychological theory and methods to patient safety.

Serwaa McClean, Patient Safety and Leadership Fellow, Bradford Institute for Health Research. Serwaa is a Specialty Trainee in Obstetrics and Gynaecology in the Yorkshire and the Humber Deanery attached to the Quality and Safety team at BIHR during an Out of Programme placement.

Naomi Quinton, Lecturer in Medical Education, Leeds Institute of Medical Education, University of Leeds. Naomi is a medical educationalist with research interests in doctors' transitions, gender in medicine, patient safety and simulation.

Penny Rhodes, Senior Research Fellow, Bradford Institute for Health Research. Penny has worked in health services research for a number of years, most recently in patient safety. She also has long-standing interests in the fields of palliative care, chronic illness, and patient and public involvement.

Valerie Rhodes, Service Improvement and Innovation Lead, Bradford District Care Trust. Val is a general/mental health nurse with considerable experience as a senior NHS manager. She worked as a fellow with the NHS Institute for Innovation and Improvement on a national health inequalities programme and currently facilitates service improvements across services within her organisation.

Victoria Robins, Patient Safety Leadership Fellow, Bradford Institute for Health Research. Victoria is a medical registrar who has worked across Yorkshire in her clinical role and as a fellowship in leadership and patient safety in pursuit of her interest in this area.

Reema Sirriyeh, Research Fellow, University of York/Bradford Institute for Health Research. Reema has a background in health psychology. She works in a joint post at the University of York and Bradford Institute for Health Research exploring the aftermath of medical error and the concept of mentorship for doctors.

Beverley Slater, Innovation and Improvement Manager, Bradford Institute for Health Research. Beverley is a psychologist and a health services manager. She has more than 10 years' experience of leading quality and safety improvement initiatives in local healthcare systems. Since March 2012 she has been Assistant Director of the Yorkshire and Humber Health Innovation and Education Cluster (HIEC) Patient Safety Theme.

Ann Starkey (MBA), Deputy Chief Executive, Medipex Ltd. Ann has over 25 years' experience of working across the boundaries of Higher Education and Healthcare Sectors. She is a Visiting Fellow at Sheffield Hallam University and a reviewer for the ESRC Knowledge Exchange Opportunities Scheme. Currently she works in operations management for Medipex Ltd.

Zoë Thompson, Lecturer in Media, Communication, Cultures, School of Cultural Studies and Humanities, Faculty of Arts, Environment and Technology, Leeds Metropolitan University. Zoë is a social scientist with particular interests in qualitative research methodologies. She has extensive experience of teaching in higher education, particularly sociology and cultural studies, at both the University of Birmingham and Leeds Metropolitan University. Her research interests include social and cultural theory, ethnography, urban regeneration and patient safety/patient involvement.

Peter Walsh, Chief Executive of Action against Medical Accidents (AvMA). Peter has extensive experience of work on patients' rights, advocacy and health policy. Before joining AvMA he was Director of the Association of Community Health Councils for England and Wales.

Jane Ward, Senior Research Fellow, Bradford Institute for Health Research. Jane is an experienced research psychologist, most recently specialising in patient involvement in patient safety and quality.

Anna Winterbottom, Senior Research Fellow, Leeds Institute for Health Sciences, University of Leeds. Anna is a research psychologist specialising in patient decision-making.

Acknowledgements

The authors and publisher would like to thank the following for permission to reproduce copyright material:

Figure 1.1 James Reason's Swiss cheese model. Adapted from Reason, JT *Managing the Risks of Organisational Accidents*, copyright 1997, with permission from Ashgate Press, Aldershot.

Figure 4.1 The system engineering initiative for patient safety (SEIPS) model of work system and patient safety. Reproduced from Work system design for patient safety: the SEIPS model, Carayon, P, Schoofs Hundt, A, Karsh, B-T, Gurses, AP, Alvarado, CJ, Smith, M and Flatley Brennan, P *Quality and Safety in Health Care*, 15 (suppl. I): i50–8, copyright 2006 with permission from BMJ Publishing Group Ltd.

Figure 4.2 Most frequently reported incident types (device-related incidents) in England and Wales from April 2006 to March 2007. Reproduced with permission from the National Patient Safety Agency, 2008.

Figure 6.4 Using PDSA (plan, do, study, act) cycles. Adapted from Langley, G, Nolan, K, Nolan, T, Norman, C and Provost, L (2009) *The Improvement Guide: A practical approach to enhancing organizational performance*, 2nd edition. San Francisco: Jossey-Bass. Copyright 2009. This material is reproduced with permission of John Wiley & Sons, Inc.

Every effort has been made to trace all copyright holders within the book, but if any have been inadvertently overlooked the publisher will be pleased to make the necessary arrangements at the first opportunity.

Introduction
Rebecca Lawton and Gerry Armitage

Keeping patients safe is an essential goal for all health professionals, and one which you must be aware of from the very beginning of your training.

Successive governments have made patient safety an NHS priority. Indeed, patient safety is not only a national priority, but a global one, as demonstrated by an increasing emphasis on the topic by the World Health Organization, which has pioneered a patient safety curriculum for undergraduate medical students (World Health Organization, 2011). Huge numbers of patients receive high-quality care from NHS staff every day. Yet statistics tell us that approximately one in every ten patients admitted to hospital is likely to suffer harm. It is no longer accepted by staff or patients that this harm is an inevitable side effect of healthcare and there is now enormous momentum for change. To change for the better requires innovators – people who are willing to do things differently or do different things. It isn't policy leaders and academics who routinely innovate for change in healthcare, but clinicians with fresh eyes and novel ideas. In this book we show you how to do this.

This book is primarily intended for undergraduate students of medicine but, as undergraduate medical students learn, and will eventually practise, within multi-disciplinary teams, this book is also of interest to all those involved in direct patient care and their managers. We believe that this book will support your learning as an undergraduate medical student. We anticipate that it will be useful during your undergraduate studies as well as following initial qualification, both as a point of reference for specific topics and as a reminder of how to improve safety and be an innovative practitioner. Unlike many of the texts you will read as a junior doctor, there is no simple answer or instruction here. Rather, we present some key issues in innovation for patient safety to guide your practice as you embark on your career in the evolving NHS. We propose that safety holds patients at the centre, and is a function of health professionals, their teams, training, education and resources. Therefore, in this book, innovation for safety is explored in a number of core areas.

The structure of this book

Throughout your reading, you will be asked to consider patient safety in its broadest sense, and to reflect on how you may develop as an innovative practitioner and an agent of change. Making an impact on patient safety is possible at every stage in your development: even as a medical undergraduate you can play a key role in influencing the safety culture and the practice within your student group.

Chapter 1 provides a foundation for many of the concepts presented in subsequent chapters. The authors consider the theories behind the patient safety movement, the policies that have made patient safety a health service priority and, as part of the same policy agenda, the need for innovation so as to improve safety. Current developments in the practice of patient safety are then highlighted, together with the challenges of changing practice.

High-quality medical education is essential to safe care. Chapter 2 reminds you of the varied and increasing opportunities for safety education as you gain more experience, and also how much patient safety impacts on your career as a junior doctor. Being safe necessitates the adoption of particular approaches to patient care. These range from being open about preventable harm or poor practice and recognition of the importance of the patient voice, to interdisciplinary working and specific communication techniques such as SBAR (situation, background, assessment, recommendation).

Chapter 3 notes the increasing momentum around involving patients in their own care in order to improve safety. It explores ways in which you might think about doing this in your own work as you embark on your medical career.

Chapter 4 explores key concepts in the field of human factors engineering for patient safety and highlights the need to recognise your limitations, and those of the technology you rely upon. The delivery of healthcare is increasingly reliant on technological support, and rapid technological innovation brings with it numerous challenges for ensuring quality and patient safety.

Chapter 5 provides an introduction to innovation in healthcare and aims to stimulate your thinking about your role in this process. The chapter includes ideas on how to be a creative and innovative practitioner as well as providing guidance on some of the tools and techniques that can help to support successful innovation.

Linked to this, Chapter 6 argues that communication and teamwork are sources of risk (and therefore safety) in healthcare. This means that there is a need for innovations to be developed and implemented by teams. This chapter presents well-tested improvement tools and case study examples to illustrate what teams can achieve when they work together to tackle safety problems.

In Chapter 7, the final chapter, we cover the topic of measurement. Whatever we do as practitioners, to improve safety (increase knowledge through training, change the equipment we use or make changes to the way we work) we need to measure the effect of these interventions on patient safety. In this chapter we explain what a good measure looks like and explore some of the challenges associated with the measurement of patient safety.

chapter 1

Introducing Patient Safety: Theory, Policy and Practice

Reema Sirriyeh, Serwaa McClean and Victoria Robins

Achieving your medical degree

This chapter will help you begin to meet the following requirements of *Tomorrow's Doctors* (General Medical Council, 2009a).

Outcome 2: The doctor as practitioner

The graduate will be able to:

17. Prescribe drugs safely, effectively and economically.

18. Carry out practical procedures safely and effectively.

Outcome 3: The doctor as professional

The graduate will be able to:

21. Reflect, learn and teach others:

   (c) Continually and systematically reflect on practice and, whenever necessary, translate that reflection into action using improvement techniques and audit appropriately – for example, by critically appraising the prescribing of others.

23. Protect patients and improve care.

   (a) Place patients' needs and safety at the centre of the care process.

Chapter overview

Patient safety is an issue that we cannot ignore. Serious errors continue to occur and conscientious, hard-working doctors can be one of the many factors that contribute to causation. The concept of learning lessons from error may seem somewhat removed from your other clinical training, yet an awareness of the safety culture and the inevitability of error is essential to reduce the chance of errors being made.

This chapter outlines prominent patient safety theory, policy and associated prac-tice. It also explores some of the main challenges to making a difference in patient safety and implementing change which you might face in your career.

After reading this chapter you will be able to discuss:

- key theoretical approaches to patient safety theory;
- the policy background and key initiatives;
- how patients can be kept safe in practice;
- challenges to implementing change in patient safety.

Introduction

For many years, medical students swore the Hippocratic oath, 'I will do no harm', at graduation. This mantra still stands strong today, yet the concept of patient safety in healthcare is relatively new. Reports such as *To Err is Human,* from the Institute of Medicine in the USA (Institute of Medicine, 1999), and its UK counterpart, *An Organisation with a Memory* (Department of Health, 2000) have fuelled a shift in government healthcare policy from quantity to quality. In 2000 the Department of Health identified the following statistics.

- 850,000 adverse healthcare events occurred in NHS hospitals every year.

- These events cost the NHS over £2bn.

- Half of them were preventable.

The preventable nature of so many of these adverse events means that trainee and junior doctors must be especially vigilant, as illustrated in the case study opposite.

DEFINITIONS

- An *adverse event* is an unintended injury caused by the healthcare system. An adverse event can occur because of things we do or things we do not do, and may or may not be preventable.
- Harm is caused when any failure within the healthcare system results in physical or psychological injury or damage.
- A *patient safety incident* (or error) refers to an unintended event caused by the healthcare system which may or may not have led to harm, and includes near-misses.

Case Study

Read the following scenario and consider the questions posed below.

A 69-year-old woman, Mrs Marsh, enters the Emergency Department (ED). She has an initial assessment by the ED junior doctor and her penicillin allergy is recorded in her medical notes but not on her wristband before she is transferred to the acute assessment unit. It is your first day on the Acute Medical Unit and you are in the middle of a consultant ward round. You are told about the penicillin allergy by the nurse who admitted Mrs Marsh. This nurse also tells you that Mrs Marsh still needs to be seen by the doctors as she has not yet been admitted to the ward due to a shortage of staff and a busy workload.

The consultant asks you to present her case but both consultant and nurse are called away to the telephone while you are doing this. On his return, the consultant tells the patient that she will be given antibiotics for a suspected chest infection and should be feeling better soon. He then leaves the room to continue the ward round. Your registrar prescribes the antibiotics according to the local guidelines. You assume that everyone is aware of the penicillin allergy and the first choice of antibiotic according to local guidelines is Augmentin, which contains penicillin.

An hour later, while you are still on the ward, a crash call is put out for help. Mrs Marsh is gasping and unable to breathe. While the team works on stabilising her, you notice that an infusion of intravenous Augmentin is running. You are unsure whether to say anything as you are a junior member of staff and are new to the ward, everyone is busy dealing with the emergency and you don't want to get your registrar in trouble. As you are about to point out that it might be an allergic reaction, the crash team leader recognises the symptoms of anaphylaxis and gives an intramuscular injection of adrenaline. Mrs Marsh quickly recovers.

Based on your reading, consider:

- What factors contributed to the adverse event described?
- What actions could have been taken to prevent this adverse event?

What might you have done differently?

A theoretical approach to patient safety

Reason's 'Swiss-cheese model'

You may be familiar with the 'Swiss-cheese model' (Figure 1.1) proposed by James Reason, a prominent psychologist and human factors expert, through which accident causation is described as the result of a series of events occurring in a sequential way.

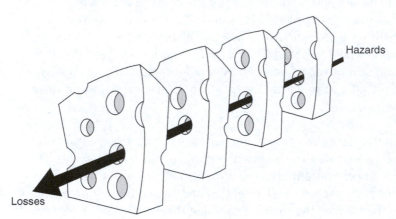

Successive layers of defences, barriers and safeguards

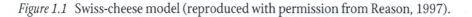

Figure 1.1 Swiss-cheese model (reproduced with permission from Reason, 1997).

Reason proposed a classification system for 'active failures' which included slips, lapses, mistakes or violations.

- A *slip* occurs when a correct action was selected but carried out incorrectly – for example, a patient's blood pressure is taken but the results are recorded in the wrong place.

- A *lapse* is the name given to a slip that results from memory failure – for example, a busy young doctor forgets that all patients presenting with a particular condition should have their blood pressure taken and omits to take it.

- A *mistake* occurs when there is a faulty plan: the individual believes the action is correct when in fact it is not. For example, a patient is wrongly diagnosed as having severe indigestion and given medication to relieve it, when in fact he is having a heart attack.

- Finally, *violations* are defined as the failure to use standard or mandatory processes (Reason, 1990). An example here might be failing to follow the standard protocol for cross-matching blood before giving a patient a transfusion.

Reason defined two further subcategories of violation: firstly, deliberate versus non-deliberate violations; and secondly, routine versus exceptional violations. Streams of patient safety literature have since emerged that focus on these different 'active failures' (Lawton, personal communication, 2011) and latent organisational failures such as understaffing, lack of staff training or faulty equipment. Such failures are described as 'latent' because they can reside unnoticed in a large organisation for long periods of time but have the capacity to be significant factors in errors at the front line of practice.

The first stream examines performance at work, focusing on changing the conditions in which humans work to enhance performance and reduce the chance of a slip, lapse or mistake occurring. The second stream of literature focuses on minimising error by targeting individuals' behaviour and reducing violations, for example through increasing adherence to organisational policy and protocol. A third stream of literature has explored the contribution of local working conditions and latent organisational failures towards error. This stream attempts to identify and target error-producing conditions, such as poor planning in the layout of drug cupboards on hospital wards.

ACTIVITY 1.1   IDENTIFYING THE HOLES

Look at the Swiss-cheese model in Figure 1.1. Do you know of an adverse event? What were the latent and active holes in that situation?

Refer back to the case study above. How would you apply Reason's Swiss-cheese model to the events described?

Other models

As a relatively new research area, theoretical models in patient safety have largely developed within the human error literature, focusing on changing systems. Human error theory (Reason, 2000) has been prominent, and proposes that human error can be understood by taking either the *person approach* or a *systems approach*. Each approach has different implications for describing error causation, and identifying the optimal approach to error management.

The person approach is focused on the unsafe acts of those at the sharp end: in healthcare this would involve a health professional making an error or violating procedure. For example, a junior doctor violates organisational policy by not recording a patient's penicillin allergy when admitting that patient to the ward. The patient then receives this drug during her stay and becomes extremely unwell. A person approach might include suspending the junior doctor until the doctor has done additional training on patient admissions.

Using this approach, an organisation attempts to manage error by reducing the variations in human behaviour that can result in mistakes; for example, by identifying those who have performed unsafe acts at the clinical front line. Improving safety following this approach would mean taking action to try and change an individual's future behaviour, for example, by attributing blame and pursuing disciplinary action. The 'person approach' and its associated management style can promote a culture of blame which can be detrimental to those at the clinical front line who may already be experiencing guilt or distress as a result of their error (Wu, 2000). On this basis, effective management of risk in healthcare is unlikely to be achieved, as learning may be hindered by health professionals' reluctance to report their own errors, or those of others, due to fear of negative personal or professional consequences (Gallagher *et al.*, 2003; Fisseni *et al.*, 2007; Scott *et al.*, 2009).

In recent years there has been a shift from person-centred error management strategies to the adoption of a systems approach, which is now the dominant paradigm in patient safety. The fundamental premise of the systems approach is that humans are fallible; therefore error is inevitable and we must be constantly vigilant. Errors are consequences, not causes and, as we cannot change human fallibility, we must change the conditions in which humans work to reduce the likelihood of error (Reason, 2000).

BOX 1.2 KEY CONCEPTS IN PATIENT SAFETY

- Errors are inevitable in a complex system such as healthcare.
- Errors within the healthcare system can be predictable and tend to repeat themselves in patterns; forgetting to record a patient's drug allergy status is not unusual in time-pressured environments.
- We should all expect and anticipate errors but do we expect to make errors in the very routine practice of prescribing antibiotics? Certain aspects of practice can facilitate *involuntary automaticity* where especially routine tasks are addressed without critical appraisal.
- Reporting clinical incidents and near-misses is the main way in which an organisation can learn and change.

Everyone has a part to play in making our systems safer. For example, the junior doctor described in the practice example may be less likely to make this type of error if the process contains appropriately targeted alerts at points where errors are more likely, and has the foresight to understand his or her own vulnerabilities in certain situations. The junior doctor may have been more vulnerable to forgetting to record allergy information because firstly, the doctor was extremely tired at the end of a long shift and secondly, he or she was recording a new and unfamiliar drug and so was focused on addressing the unfamiliar drug rather than attending to screening and recording drug allergies. By recognising the clinician's own limitations (tiredness) and the risks of attentional bias (focusing on the unfamiliar drug), the junior doctor could reduce the likelihood of making this mistake.

The concept of the systems approach originated in high-risk, high-reliability industries such as aviation (Helmreich, 2000) and the petrochemical industries. This approach offers a useful and arguably more effective strategy for understanding and identifying risks in a complex work environment where teams and technology interact. The associated risk management strategies attempt to build defences in the local work environment, and at an organisational level, to prevent or reduce error likelihood.

One example of a strategy to minimise the risk of error using a systems approach is storing similar-sounding or looking drugs separately, or changing the packaging to make the different drugs distinctive. This reduces the chance of the wrong drug being given. Reason (2000) proposed that, by recognising and accepting human variability and approaching error management in this way, organisations can devote management resources to a more comprehensive approach that takes into account individuals, teams, local conditions and latent organisational failures. By adopting this approach, organisations might also be able to move away from a culture of fear that focuses on attributing blame and individual culpability towards a more posi-tive reporting culture around risk and a safer workplace. Importantly, the systems approach acknowledges that decisions by those at the 'blunt end' of the system (e.g. managers, clinical governance leads) about budgeting, planning and staffing policy are central to the safety culture that is created. Poor decisions at the blunt end can result in latent organisational error, and the creation of error-producing conditions, in which human performance by frontline staff is prone to failure (Reason, 2000).

Reason's work has been extremely influential in the development of quality and safety policy in the UK and further afield. The Department of Health's strategic approach to patient safety is underpinned by the systems approach; policy docu-ments consistently refer to the need to promote organisational defences, and to acknowledge the role of systems issues in patient safety. Key pieces of patient safety policy, which have a direct bearing on your day-to-day working life as a doctor, are overviewed in the following section.

A policy approach to patient safety

Unlike the theory literature, policy documents have largely evolved from the second stream of patient safety literature and largely focused on promoting safer practice by developing rules and guidelines and encouraging people to comply with them. Recent policy documents have been a driving force in attempts to change the culture of healthcare.

A policy of change

Lord Darzi's final report of his NHS *Next Stage Review* (Department of Health, 2008) redefined the purpose of the NHS. Darzi proposed that regulation should no longer be its organising principle, but that clinical effectiveness, patient safety and patient experience, under the umbrella of quality, should take its place. Darzi aimed to foster the development of clinical leaders managing services at a local level and to promote greater patient empowerment.

A culture of innovation in which new ideas, technologies and processes are con-stantly developed, evaluated and refined was described as central to ensuring con-tinuous improvement in care quality. Many innovations come from staff working in the health service and the government are keen to encourage the next generation of health professionals to evolve as innovative practitioners. New partnerships between the NHS, universities and industry have been established in the drive to encourage innovation and ongoing development via research, along with an independent Innovation Fund, and a series of Health Innovation and Education Clusters (HIECs).

ACTIVITY 1.2

When leaders begin to change their responses to mistakes and failure, asking what happened instead of who made the error, the culture within healthcare institutions will begin to change.

(Botwinick *et al.*, 2006)

In *High Quality Care for All: NHS next stage review* (Department of Health, 2008), Lord Darzi encouraged clinicians to be practitioners, partners and leaders in the NHS. Thinking about the quotation above and with reference to both the *Leadership Guide to Patient Safety* and the Darzi Report, consider what leadership in healthcare means to you and how it might influence patient safety.

- What examples have you seen in practice of good and poor leadership?
- What leadership behaviours might be important for you to develop that would influence safety practices within the teams you are in?

The Darzi Report (Department of Health, 2008) paved the way for a major cultural shift in the NHS, which has implications for you as the next generation of doctors. Change in the NHS will require doctors not only to have excellent clinical skills and knowledge, but also to be effective and accountable clinical leaders. There is a growing demand for doctors to:

- reject long-standing professional boundaries;
- reflect on current practice;
- engage in new ways of thinking;
- work as innovative practitioners in multidisciplinary teams.

Innovative practice with which you might become directly involved could include:

- identifying new ways to engage patients in their own care (Chapter 3);
- embedding research and development into care across your clinical team (Chapter 6);
- making use of novel technology and knowledge to enhance care quality and safety (Chapter 4).

In 2010, the White Paper *Equity and Excellence: Liberating the NHS* (Department of Health, 2010a) set out a strategy for major reform and transformation of healthcare provision in the UK, laying out plans to:

- abolish primary care trusts and strategic health authorities;

- create around 500 general practitioner consortia responsible for healthcare commissioning (deciding how to distribute NHS funds);

- pass public health duties to local authorities;

- allow all NHS providers to become foundation trusts;

- make changes to healthcare regulation.

With regard to the last point, changes in healthcare regulation have been limited to date, as responsibilities for the regulation of quality (Care Quality Commission) and for the regulation of finance (Monitor) remain distinct. In addition to the changes described, the Department of Health is losing many of its functions to an independent NHS board. These dramatic changes will have major implications for all those who work within the NHS and for the general public who use the service. The key messages delivered through this paper are that responsibility should be devolved to clinical and local leaders and high-quality care must come from focusing on outcomes and empowering patients.

The Quality, Innovation, Productivity and Prevention Programme (QIPP) was introduced in response to the government White Paper and is an attempt to challenge the NHS workforce to use innovation as a way of delivering high-quality, safe care within ever-tightening budgetary limitations. In the programme, the Department of Health sets out three reasons why innovation is important, and what kinds of things we can do to promote innovation in the NHS (see 'What's the evidence?').

What's the evidence?

1. *Innovation improves and extends lives. Innovation in the NHS is about making a real and tangible difference to the lives of millions. Across the NHS, countless patients bear witness to the power of great ideas.*

   One of the drivers behind the reformation of the NHS is to reduce bureaucracy and barriers to innovation and give clinicians with the knowledge and skills the opportunity to develop ideas and interventions and the autonomy to put these into practice. Innovation can increase quality and productivity, for example by reducing patient waiting lists or decreasing the length of hospital stays after surgery. Innovations are not always costly and may often simplify procedures and cut costs.

2. *Innovation connects and drives quality and productivity in the NHS. The NHS faces a challenging future with increasing financial pressures and continually increasing demand for improved quality of services. It is clear that the NHS must raise its game to develop more high-quality and cost-effective interventions if it is to keep improving.*

By putting patients at the centre and focusing and tailoring care to individual needs, we can create better services, streamline efficiency and reduce waste. One example of integrating systems to improve quality and productivity is providing more care in the community for patients with chronic diseases. This may improve their quality of life, while releasing hospital beds and reducing the risk of hospital acquired infections. Promoting care in the community may also decrease costs associated with patient transport, lost days at work and childcare.

3. *Innovation will support the UK economy. The NHS remains a major investor and wealth creator in the UK, and in science and engineering in particular. Innovation is not just about the future of the NHS and health and social care, it is about the future of our country's economy too.*

How can the NHS boost our economy? Andrew Lansley (2011) drew attention to the fact that the NHS is a major source of income, providing consultancy and sharing expertise worldwide. It also sells services – for example, Moorfield Eye Hospital runs a clinic in Dubai generating large revenue that is reinvested in the NHS. Great Ormond Street Hospital is also renowned worldwide for its excellent services, and because of this has many private patients who also generate finance (Lansley, 2011).

Accountability and governance

Since 2010, healthcare institutions have been required to publish quality accounts in addition to their finances, and this has meant that priorities in healthcare have changed. These documents delivered a clear and stark message to politicians, healthcare providers and, importantly, to the general public: healthcare is not as safe as it could be, errors are inevitable and more could be done to improve safety. An explosion of interest in exploring and improving patient safety has resulted, as evidenced by the establishment of the National Patient Safety Agency in 2003 in the UK and the Center for Quality and Improvement in Patient Safety in 2004 in the USA. Safe healthcare is not solely reliant on expert health professionals adhering to best clinical practice. Safety must be built into systems, through well-designed care structures and processes and backed by substantial organisational support.

Innovation can sometimes be a slow process from idea to actuation, and there is a drive to increase the ease with which innovations can be developed, refined, adopted and spread, so that innovation and growth are ongoing and embedded in the NHS (Department of Health, 2011a). In the following section, we explore how policy has been translated into practice, by discussing recent innovations in patient safety which have been enacted at national and local level through patient safety initiatives and campaigns.

Patient safety in practice

Patient Safety First was launched nationally in 2008 as a two-year-long patient safety campaign, with the aim of facilitating a cultural shift and behavioural change with regard to safety in NHS organisations. The campaign focused on five interventions that were consistently identified in prior research as having a significant impact on patient safety. Each trust was invited to participate voluntarily, firstly in the leadership intervention and then to choose how many of the other four interventions they wished to engage in. The interventions were as follows.

1. leadership for safety, which focused on getting executive boards fully engaged and demonstrating that patient safety was their highest priority;

2. reducing harm from deterioration, i.e. early recognition and treatment of the deteriorating patient;

3. reducing harm in critical care, i.e. reducing infections from central lines and ventilator-associated pneumonia;

4. reducing harm in perioperative care, i.e. reducing surgical site infections and implementation of the World Health Organization surgical checklist;

5. reducing harm from high-risk medicines, i.e. reducing harm associated with anti-coagulants, injectable sedatives, opiates and insulin.

Local initiatives

Local safety initiatives are also common. For example, the SAFE! campaign was a locally run initiative in a Yorkshire trust that identified strategies to combat a range of safety issues. Each patient safety issue was addressed with a separate intervention on a month-by-month basis, e.g. one month the focus was on modified early warnings scores (MEWS) that use four physiological markers (systolic blood pressure, heart rate, body temperature and respiratory rate) and one observational marker (level of consciousness) to identify deteriorating patients. Changes in the composite score can act as a trigger for health professionals to escalate their response, as described in the case study below.

Case study

A 19-year-old woman is admitted to hospital with abdominal pain and query appendicitis. The medical team decide to adopt a watch-and-wait approach, observing her before deciding what action should be taken. The woman is observed by a healthcare assistant who regularly checks on her but does not tabulate her MEWS score. After some time the patient is transferred to another ward, but her observations are lost in the transfer process. She arrests on the new ward and in the subsequent case review it is revealed that her initial MEWS score was noted as 5 but that no medical opinion was sought and her care was not escalated as a result.

All clinical staff were educated about MEWS and required to pass a competency assessment, resulting in significant improvements in recording and acting on patients' observations. The campaign was marketed throughout the trust and accompanied by spot checks and audits, with the results publicised internally so departments could analyse their progress.

Such initiatives have had varying degrees of success. Some of the main difficulties experienced are:

- finding accurate measures to assess changes in safety attitudes and behaviours (Chapter 7)
- ensuring that information is effectively cascaded to those on the clinical front line, i.e. the people who have direct patient contact.

The challenge of reaching front-line staff through such initiatives was recognised in the Patient Safety First campaign. One approach to address this was using the personal narratives of individuals' achievements within the participating trusts to inspire people to act.

ACTIVITY 1.3

Look up the Patient Safety First website (**www.patientsafetyfirst.nhs.uk**). Using the interventions tab, consider what types of interventions might be introduced to your clinical area that could enhance patient safety.

Although successful campaigns rely on senior management support to drive them and identify what is permissible and feasible from an organisational viewpoint, practitioners on the shop floor who are responsible for implementing change must have some ownership (Greenfield *et al.*, 2011). Innovations from staff working on the front line also benefit from their knowledge and understanding of the tasks they carry out on a daily basis.

Patient experience

Historically the healthcare system functioned on the old adage that 'doctor knows best' – doctors are experts, and not to be questioned. This culture is changing rapidly and, as the public demand more choice and input into their care, patients are no longer expected to be passive recipients of care, but active partners. The delivery of healthcare ultimately affects patients' lives; therefore, they have the ethical and moral right to be involved in decision-making processes, and to access information and question health professionals about their care. As knowledge of patient safety grows, there is a greater appreciation of the value of involving patients in their care (Department of Health, 2005, 2008, 2010a; Koutantji *et al.*, 2005; Ward and Armitage, 2012). Patients now have increased access to healthcare information and engaging patients in decision-making helps to ensure that policies and practices reflect their needs and preferences (International Alliance of Patient Organisations, 2005). Promoting patients' responsibility for their own care might also result in optimal usage of the healthcare system, leading to improved health outcomes, quality of life and patient satisfaction, while reducing costs. For more information on involving patients in their own safety, see Chapter 3.

Developing leadership attributes in doctors

As a doctor you have an intrinsic leadership role within healthcare. Your behaviour and decisions have both direct and long-term consequences for your patients, and for your team. Despite your rapidly changing and complex work environment, you are often held accountable for your actions and, if something goes wrong (for example, a patient is prescribed the wrong dose of a harmful drug), you will experience scrutiny from colleagues, patients and their families, perhaps local communities and even the mass media. A similar level of scrutiny might also occur from simply changing an aspect of clinical practice; for example, the implementation of a new handover strategy to address problems you have identified in your ward may not be welcomed by other team members who are happy with the current approach. One of the key points made in the Darzi Report was that making change actually happen takes leadership, and is central to our expectations of the healthcare professionals of tomorrow (Department of Health, 2008). You will be expected to make a contribution to the effective running of the organisation in which you work, and have a responsibility to drive up standards of patient safety. This position brings with it the chance to make a real difference in healthcare, but to do this you will be expected to develop skills to guide, influence and motivate the safety attitudes and practices of your team.

The challenges of implementing change in patient safety

Despite the widespread recognition of patient safety concerns, and a desire to address these through innovation, there has been limited success in implementing such change in the health service. The development of patient safety solutions is often a challenging and time-consuming process, with the effectiveness of resulting interventions difficult to ascertain. There are many reasons for the slow progress of change; Leistikow *et al.* (2011) recently proposed four key challenges in patient safety work: visibility, ambiguity, complexity and autonomy.

Visibility

Patient safety issues are often not readily visible in healthcare, in comparison to other competing demands on service providers. Patient safety issues are often only discovered when a serious adverse event occurs, which is followed by a systematic investigation. Often, the scale of unsafe practice is not easily recognised by organisational leaders to enable them to justify the dedication of organisational resources to these; for example, many junior doctors might experience challenges undertaking their daily ward rounds with a senior colleague, but the safety risk that this creates may go unnoticed until a mistake is made.

Ambiguity

In addition, there is ambiguity in identifying what a patient safety issue is, and what type of solution is required. It may often be difficult to determine the precise cause of a death or delayed hospital stay, and to be certain that this occurred as the result of an error or violation, particularly when dealing with patients in very poor health. Furthermore, attributing the cause of error more broadly as either the result of an individual's unsafe act or as a systems failing can be difficult. Despite a shift towards the systems approach, Leistikow and colleagues (2011) highlight that in many cases there is an argument for attributing a patient safety incident to both individual and systems failings. Woods and Cook (2002) highlight the intrinsic role of individuals in creating safety, which reinforces the challenges of separating individual and systems failings in the event of an error. For example, an individual doctor may prescribe the incorrect dose of Clexane to a patient, and that individual action puts the patient at risk; however, if there is a shortage of staff due to poor planning and a lack of financial resource, the doctor may have too many patients to see, which has caused that doctor to rush and was a major contributor to this mistake.

Complexity

The provision of healthcare is extremely complex, and this creates major challenges for patient safety interventions. Multiple features of the 'tightly coupled' processes (Perrow, 1984) in healthcare have an influence on patient safety, including the immediate structure of the workplace, equipment available, organisational protocols, time of day and the knowledge and skills of health professionals. It may seem impossible to account for this multitude of factors when developing a safety solution. It can also be difficult to reach a consensus about which patient safety issue to prioritise, and how to explore it in such a complex environment. As an example, is it more useful to dedicate resources to training staff to reduce the chance of patient safety incidents occurring at an organisation-wide level, or should resources be dedicated to addressing problems in specific wards which relate to a particular threat, such as the confusion caused by variations in handover procedures (handover board, paper-based or electronic systems) from ward to ward?

Autonomy

The fourth and final challenge raised by Leistikow and colleagues (2011) is that of autonomy. It is essential for doctors to have some degree of autonomy in their role to make the most appropriate decisions based on their knowledge and skill. However, a consequence of protecting autonomy is the development of a culture of non-intervention, in which it can often be considered inappropriate to challenge the actions of a colleague, even when this may protect patients. In a sample of 1,318 doctors, around 50 per cent expressed difficulty in challenging colleagues about their practice, including highlighting an unsafe act (Aasland and Forde, 2005). In a culture of non-intervention, the imposition of a patient safety solution can be perceived as an unwelcome intervention which threatens autonomy, and is therefore poorly received. For example, the introduction of a buddying system as a point of contact and support for new specialist trainees in a trust might actually be perceived as the trust suggesting that they are incompetent and therefore these trainees may avoid contact with their buddy, resulting in an ineffective intervention.

Many additional factors can stunt the implementation of patient safety interventions. There can be great variation in the safety culture of different subgroups within a single organisation; therefore staff in one clinical or professional group may be more receptive to a particular safety solution than those in another. The discussion of error and risk can be challenging in many healthcare settings, which can make it difficult to identify and address such problems. It is important to recognise and account for these types of barrier where possible when considering how you may pursue your own patient safety interventions, particularly when there is change and uncertainty and resources are limited. There are several ways this can be approached, but in the first instance, simply considering the environment in which a patient safety solution will operate and recognising where possible barriers may lie may be helpful. Important issues to consider include how you can provide evidence that a problem exists requiring a patient safety solution and how you can measure the impact of the solution to demonstrate its effectiveness subsequently. It is also important to develop a culture where anyone who recognises a breach in safety feels able to speak out, as the case study below illustrates.

Case Study: Exposing patients to infection

Staff seeing patients on the wards of a district general hospital were complying with most infection control policies.

- They washed their hands properly between patients.
- They didn't wear ties.
- They didn't sit on beds.

Despite this, there was an outbreak of *Staphylococcus aureus* on the ward.

- How could this have happened?

It was a student who noticed that the doctors were not cleaning their stethoscopes between patients. On examination, all the stethoscopes were found to be carrying *S. aureus*.

• How could cross-infection be prevented?

The student suggested putting stethoscope-cleaning equipment by the sink where the staff washed their hands in the ward. Repeat random swabbing of the stethoscopes showed that they were no longer contaminated with *S. aureus*.

Consider:

• If you had been the student in this situation, would you have been so observant?
• Would you have had the courage to speak up and challenge the practice of senior colleagues?
• Would you have had the imagination and the confidence to suggest a remedy?

As one of tomorrow's doctors, you have a duty to do everything in your power to keep patients safe.

Chapter summary

In this chapter, you have been introduced to key theoretical concepts in patient safety research and relevant patient safety policies. The role of recent policy documents and their translation into practice have been illustrated by a discussion of recent initiatives, campaigns and educational developments. We have looked at some of the barriers to patient safety, and suggested some ways that these might be overcome.

GOING FURTHER

To find out more about the UK policy agenda, see the following documents:

Department of Health (2005) *Creating a Patient-led NHS: Delivering the NHS improvement plan*. London: Department of Health.

Department of Health (2008) *Next Stage Review: High quality healthcare for all*. London: Department of Health.

Department of Health (2010) *Equity and Equality: Liberating the NHS*. London: Department of Health.

The following article gives a more detailed discussion of patients' involvement in their own safety:

Koutantji, M, Davis, R, Vincent, CA and Coulter, A (2005) The patient's role in patient safety: engaging patients, their representatives, and health professionals. *Clinical Risk*, 11: 99–104.

For further discussion of the challenges in implementing patient safety, see:

Leistikow, I, Kalkman, CJ and Bruijn, H (2011) Why patient safety is such a tough nut to crack. *British Medical Journal*, 342: d3447.

The websites below give more information about using innovative approaches to address patient safety problems:

Patient Safety First (2008) **www.patientsafetyfirst.nhs.uk/ashx/Asset. ashx?path=/Patient%20Safety%20First%20-%20the%20campaign %20review.pdf.**

Quality, Innovation, Production, Prevention (QIPP) **www.institute.nhs.uk/cost_ and_quality/qipp/cost_and_quality_homepage.html.**

To find out more about the theoretical models discussed in this chapter, see:

Reason, J (1990) *Human Error*. New York: Cambridge University Press.

Reason, J (2000) Human error: models and management. *British Medical Journal*, 320 (7237): 768.

chapter 2

Enhancing Your Learning for Patient Safety

Naomi Quinton, Zoë Thompson,
Anna Winterbottom and Vikram Jha

Achieving your medical degree

This chapter will help you to meet the following requirements of *Tomorrow's Doctors* (General Medical Council, 2009a) and the *Foundation Programme Curriculum* (Department of Health, 2011b).

Outcome 3: The doctor as a professional

The graduate will be able to:

23. Protect patients and improve care:

   (d) Promote, monitor and maintain health and safety in the clinical setting, understanding how errors can happen in practice, applying the principles of quality assurance, clinical governance and risk management to medical practice, and understanding responsibilities within the current systems for raising concerns about safety and quality.

   (e) Understand and have experience of the principles and methods of improvement, including audit, adverse incident reporting and quality improvement, and how to use the results of audit to improve practice.

   (f) Respond constructively to the outcomes of appraisals, performance reviews and assessments.

Focus on patient safety within the Foundation Programme Curriculum

7. Patient safety within clinical governance

Outcome: demonstrates a clear commitment to maintaining patient safety and delivering high-quality reliable care. Understand that clinical governance is the over-arching framework that unites a range of quality improvement activities to safeguard standards and facilitate improvements in clinical services.

7.1. Treats the patient as the centre of care

Competences

- listens actively and enables patients to express concerns and preferences, ask questions and make personal choices
- respects the right to autonomy and confidentiality
- recognises the patient's confidence and competence to self-care and need for support, notably when an acute problem is superimposed on a chronic illness
- seeks advice promptly when unable to answer a patient's query or concerns
- respects the patient's right to refuse treatment or take part in research
- considers care pathways and the process of care from the patient's perspective
- describes common reactions of patients, family and clinical staff to error
- places the needs of patients above own convenience without compromising the safety of self or others.

7.2. Makes patient safety a priority in own clinical practice

Competences

- identifies and minimises potential risks and main hazards to patients
- delivers protocol-driven care
- describes a critical incident and methods of preventing an adverse event
- identifies or describes a potential complaint and the role of the multidisciplinary team in methods of resolution
- provides reliable best practice care based on clinical care pathways, care bundles or protocols
- maintains professional development to enhance personal contribution to quality of patient care.

7.3. Promotes patient safety through good team working

Competences

- works in partnership with patients and colleagues to develop sustainable care plans to manage patients' acute and chronic conditions
- cross-checks instructions and actions with colleagues, e.g. medicines to be injected
- draws attention to risks or potential risks to patients regardless of status of colleagues
- describes ways of identifying and dealing with poor performance in self and colleagues, including senior colleagues.

7.4. Understands the principles of quality and safety improvement

Competences

- demonstrates knowledge of how and when to report adverse events and 'near misses' to local and, where appropriate, national reporting systems.

- describes opportunities for improving the reliability of care following adverse events or 'near misses'
- describes root-cause analysis.

7.5. Complaints

Competences

- is sensitive to situations where patients are unhappy with aspects of care and seeks to remedy concerns with help from senior colleagues and/or other members of the multidisciplinary team
- always behaves in a way that appropriately minimises the risk of causing patient dissatisfaction.

Chapter overview

Learning about patient safety is an essential part of your medical training and your ongoing practice. This chapter will help you understand where within your curriculum, or in more informal settings, you currently have the opportunity to learn about patient safety. It will also provide you with tools to help you work within your capabilities, appropriate to your stage of development, and suggest methods of challenging appropriately when you have concerns about unsafe practice. Patient safety is a feature at every stage in your training, and something you should be constantly aware of regardless of the stage you are at or the specialty you choose.

After reading this chapter, you will be able to:

- explain why patient safety is so important to medical students and Foundation doctors and be able to describe your appreciation of the current professional guidelines on patient safety;
- demonstrate your ability to recognise the different contexts for learning about patient safety (formal and informal);
- explore how learning opportunities will help you become a safer practitioner;
- discuss innovations in patient safety training.

Introduction: Why is patient safety important for you as a medical student or trainee doctor?

Ten per cent of all hospital admissions in the UK result in an adverse event for patients. Approximately ten per cent of these adverse events result in death (De Vries *et al.*, 2008). That means, that for every 100 admissions, one patient dies from an incident not directly related to his or her admission, but directly related to treatment or the healthcare system.

Given these startling figures, you can see why you need to learn how to practise as safely as possible. Practising safely is at the core of being a 'good' doctor. Your patients and their safety should be at the centre of your practice.

As a medical student or trainee you are responsible for *ensuring patient safety by working within the limits of your competence, training and status* and for *raising any concerns about patient safety or any aspect of the conduct of others which is inconsistent with good professional practice* (General Medical Council, 2009a, p13). The *Foundation Programme Curriculum* (Department of Health, 2011b) makes it clear that ensuring patient safety is a core part of your learning, and an area in which you must demonstrate competence across five different fields, as shown above.

This chapter presents you with a range of options to enhance your ability to recognise learning opportunities in patient safety and the different contexts for learning. It also introduces you, through a series of case studies, to innovative practices in patient safety training.

Finally, it demonstrates why patient safety is best thought of as something that is fundamental to all aspects of clinical practice, from history-taking and patient interactions to prescribing and administering medicines. In other words, a good doctor is one who practises safely.

'Just a routine operation'

Unacceptable numbers of patients are harmed as a result of their treatment or as a consequence of their admission to hospital. One such patient was Elaine Bromley.

Watch the video 'Just a routine operation', at: **www.institute.nhs.uk/safer_care/general/human_factors.html.**

What do you think happened in this situation? What elements acted together to cause this avoidable event?

Discussion

On the surface this appears to be a tragic but unavoidable event resulting from an unexpected but recognised complication of anaesthesia. The outcome might have been very different if the team had an awareness of human factors and how these affect performance of people and teams under stress. All team members treating Elaine were very experienced and competent, yet a series of unforeseen events led to her death. The investigation into her death highlighted the following contributory factors.

- A loss of situational awareness – in a stressful situation, the consultants became focused on one factor, inserting the breathing tube and losing sight of the bigger picture.
- Perception and cognition – the actions of members of the team were not aligned with their emergency protocols and may not have been the best option.

- Teamwork – there was no clear leader, which led to a breakdown in the decision-making process.
- Culture – nurses sensed the urgency but did not raise their concerns aloud. The hierarchy of the team made assertiveness difficult despite the severity of the situation.

DEFINITION

Human factors encompass all those factors that can influence people and their behaviour. In a work context, human factors are the environmental, organisational and job factors and individual characteristics that influence behaviour at work (Carthey and Clarke, 2009).

You can read more about human factors in patient safety at: **www.institute.nhs. uk/images//documents/SaferCare/Human-Factors-How-to-Guide-v1.2.pdf**.

Types of learning

Learning about patient safety takes place at the level of the individual, the curriculum within which healthcare professionals study and the organisation in which they are placed – for example, a hospital ward, a GP practice or in the class-room. You, as a learner, need to take responsibility for your own learning and prac-tice and remember that during your training you will be working within a system that brings different opportunities to different people. For example, during your training you have the opportunity to experience a variety of healthcare settings in your placements. It is important that you consider the value of each opportunity from the clinical teaching to the patients you meet as a resource for improving your practice of patient safety. You will need to be able to recognise when and how learn-ing about patient safety might take place. Not only will this enable you to fulfil the requirements of your course, it will also help you to live up to the expectation that medical students and trainees are the clinical leaders of the future. Effective leader-ship is a vital component of patient safety since a clinical team takes direction from the team leader's attitude and behaviour (Mohr *et al.*, 2002). A safe leader encour-ages a safe team.

The opportunities to learn about patient safety during your training may not always be obvious. For example, during a placement you may have been party to a conversation about how certain processes or clinical pathways are followed; perhaps you have discussed a specific antibiotic-prescribing protocol that is utilised within a certain ward. This section demonstrates how patient safety is incorporated as a central theme in your undergraduate medical curriculum and initial training and how you can maximise your ability to access these learning opportunities.

ACTIVITY 2.1 PEER-TO-PEER LEARNING

Look closely at the criteria laid out by *Tomorrow's Doctors* (General Medical Council, 2009a), and at the Foundation Years curriculum for your university. Which of these aspects of patient safety have you encountered as part of your training? To what extent have you experienced them in clinical practice (while on placement, for example)?

Cross-reference this with the experience of a peer from the same or another university. How does your perceived learning to date about patient safety differ?

Discuss whether, on the basis of your experience so far, you feel confident about your ability to practise safely and consider what you might do to improve your awareness in this area.

Formal learning about patient safety

Undergraduate medical degrees differ in the extent to which they have an explicit patient safety theme. At the University of Leeds, for example, the recently introduced MB ChB curriculum, *Curriculum 2010*, has patient safety teaching at the heart of a mandatory longitudinal strand which students in all their years of training have to complete. Here, patient safety deliberately sits alongside other core elements of good clinical practice, including leadership, professionalism and team working, to emphasise that patient safety is a holistic concept which is intrinsic to all types of professional behaviour that doctors engage in. Patient safety themes are revisited at various points throughout the course, with increasing complexity. In Liverpool Medical School, there is a specific module that emphasises patient safety in the final year of the curriculum. This is designed so students build the necessary confidence in various clinical skills that are often related to patient safety incidents, for example, safe prescribing. This allows new doctors to 'hit the ground running' in their Foundation year. Both of these approaches are in line with the emergent international curriculum framework for safety education and training developed from the Australian Safety and Quality Council (World Health Organization, 2009).

What are the priorities for patient safety?

World Health Organization curriculum on patient safety

The World Health Organization determined that healthcare students and newly qualified professionals need to know how systems impact on the quality and safety of care, how poor communication may lead to adverse events and how to manage these challenges in their daily practice. This led to the publication of their multiprofessional patient safety curriculum guide.

- What is patient safety?
- What are human factors and why are they important for patient safety?
- Understanding systems and the impact of complexity on patient care;
- Being an effective team player;
- Understanding and learning from errors;
- Understanding and managing clinical risk;
- Introduction to quality improvement methods;
- Engaging with patients and carers;
- Minimising infection through improved infection control;
- Patient safety and invasive procedures;
- Improving medication safety.

You can read more about the development of the curricula and why each item was included, along with case studies and exercises, at: **www.who.int/patientsafety/education/curriculum/en/index.html**.

Why should the factors outlined in the box above be pertinent to teaching about patient safety? We understand from work by the National Patient Safety Agency (NPSA) how team factors and problems with communication are a common cause of all error types and how medication errors contribute to patient safety incidents (Cousins, 2007). This work by the NPSA has led to providing case studies which can be used for all healthcare professionals to learn about enhancing patient safety.

An example of formal teaching about patient safety from the first year of the Leeds medical school curriculum concerns the death of a patient due to medical error. In this case, the removal of the patient's healthy kidney left him with only one non-functioning kidney. During the court investigation it was noted that, prior to the removal of the healthy kidney, a medical student who was observing the operation voiced concern that an error was about to occur. Unfortunately, she was ignored by the medical team, with disastrous consequences. Part of your duty as a medical student is to speak up about any threats to patient safety, even under difficult or challenging circumstances. Despite the adverse outcome for the patient the medical

ACTIVITY 2.2

Think about how you would have reacted if you had observed that operation.

What are the ways in which you might have challenged constructively while making yourself heard? Would you demand that the operation be stopped? How might you continue to challenge even after rebuttal when you know you are right? With a peer, allocate yourselves the role of junior and senior colleagues.

Using the example of the kidney operation above, practise some phrases of increasing severity that might help you raise the alarm to colleagues. Make a note of these and then switch roles. Between you, agree a set of phrases you feel would be effective at challenging the actions of senior colleagues. Perhaps you could initiate the PACE tool for assertiveness, as described below.

Note

It is now common practice in UK operating theatres to have a 'time out' before starting an operation as well as a team briefing before the theatre list start. This is so that all team members are ready to anticipate problems and are aware of what kit will be required. Each member of the team has to confirm that they agree it is the correct patient, the correct procedure and the correct site before surgery starts. If the patient is having local anaesthesia, he or she has to agree as well! This practice was introduced because analysis of cases of 'wrong-site surgery' showed that, in nearly every case, there was someone in theatre who knew it was the wrong site, but did not feel able to speak up. Never be afraid to state the obvious.

student in this case acted responsibly and correctly.

A useful method of helping you challenge patient safety issues is to adopt the PACE graded assertiveness tool. This model was adopted from the aviation industry where it was discovered that pilots were concerned about challenging authority (Besco, 1999). The Tenerife runway disaster in 1977, involving a runway collision between Pan American flight 1736 and KLM flight 4805, is the accident with the highest number of fatalities in aviation history, with 583 people killed. The investigation that followed found that the accident was the result of communication failure and, in particular, the failure to challenge seniority. The accident investigator reported that the first officer in one of the planes had found it difficult to challenge the well-respected and experienced pilot prior to the collision (Krause, 2003).

Commentators have noted that the issue of challenging authority is equally relevant in medicine, given its hierarchical nature, which can hamper good communication. Previous research has identified that this problem is most commonly seen between doctors and nurses but it is equally relevant between other healthcare professionals and between doctors at different levels of seniority (Porter and Samovar, 1991; Sweet and Norman, 1995; Fagin and Garelick, 2004). Given this, graded assertiveness is a useful tool for the medical profession too (Attree, 2007; Chiarella and McInnes, 2008). The main priority of graded assertiveness is to communicate clearly and concisely your concerns in a way that prioritises the patient's safety rather than protecting the ego of the senior clinician (Hunt *et al.*, 2007). As Curtis *et al.* (2011) point out, your role here is vital and concerns your status as the patient's advocate.

The key stages of graded assertiveness indicated by the acronym PACE are given in the box below.

PACE

- *Probe*   'Do you know that . . .?'
- *Alert*   'Can we reassess the situation . . .?'
- *Challenge*   'Please stop what you are doing for a minute while . . .'
- *Emergency!* 'Stop what you are doing!'

If we consider the example above of wrong-site surgery, where the wrong kidney was removed, we could use the PACE graded assertiveness tool as follows.

- *Probe*   'Do you know that this might be the wrong kidney?'
- *Alert*   'Can we reassess the situation and check that we're concentrating on the correct kidney?'
- *Challenge*   'Please stop what you are doing for a minute while we check we're about to remove the correct kidney.'
- *Emergency!* 'Stop what you are doing! This is the wrong kidney.'

Learning point

You are now better equipped to understand the formal contexts in which you might learn about patient safety as a medical student or Foundation trainee and how to work alongside your peers to improve your learning.

Informal learning about patient safety

During your training, you will undertake a series of placements in different clinical environments. This will involve you interacting with a range of other healthcare professionals and with patients in both formal and informal ways. As a junior doctor, you will find yourself influenced by the behaviour and practices of a number of senior colleagues, including consultants and senior nurses. Most of the time, you will find that their behaviour reflects good practice with regard to patient safety. You will find, for instance, that there are protocols and guidelines on the wards to which these people refer when managing patients. You will also see them maintaining hygiene, e.g. hand-washing, and other activities such as cross-checking prescriptions, asking for help from colleagues when in doubt. These are all examples of positive role modelling.

On occasions, however, you may find that some senior colleagues deliberately do not adhere to some protocols. This does not mean that they are necessarily unsafe practitioners. It is usually because these people can use their experience to make informed judgments on whether or not to follow guidelines strictly. It is also often the case that, once you are on placement, in a real clinical environment, much of your theoretical knowledge of patient safety might be challenged by, for example, time pressures or the local culture of 'how things are done around here'. However, if you think that the safety of patients is at risk, then it is your duty to ask for support or question the local practice. Assurance that patient safety is being maintained, and an explanation of how it is being maintained, is essential.

ACTIVITY 2.3 REFLECTION

On your next placement, make a point of observing how doctors communicate with other doctors and healthcare professionals. What kinds of information need to be communicated to ensure the safety of the patient?

Think about examples of good and poor communication that you have witnessed during your clinical experience. List the key features of each.

One way in which you can ensure that the correct information is communicated in order to ensure patient safety is to use the SBARR (situation, background, assessment, recommendation, readback) tool. This standardised tool helps practitioners to communicate all the relevant information to colleagues (for example, when requesting help from a senior colleague) and to patients and their families. Like the PACE tool, other industries such as the military and aviation have offered useful methods to develop and improve communication skills (Helmreich, 2000). SBARR was originally developed for the US Navy but refined for use in healthcare settings by patient safety expert Michael Leonard and his colleagues at Kaiser Permanente in Colorado, USA. Given that communication failures are a common cause of adverse patient incidents, standardising certain aspects of communication is a key strategy in both encouraging effective teamwork and reducing risk to patients (Leonard *et al.*, 2004).

SBARR

S Situation

- Identify yourself and the site/unit you are calling from.
- Identify the patient by name and the reason for your report.
- Describe your concern.

B Background

- Give the patient's reason for admission.
- Explain significant medical history.
- You then inform your colleague of the patient's background: diagnosis on admission, date of admission, prior medical/surgical procedures, current medications, allergies, pertinent laboratory results and other relevant diagnostic results. For this, you need to have collected information from the patient's chart, flow sheets and progress notes.

A Assessment

Assess:

- vital signs;
- contraction pattern;
- clinical impressions, concerns.

You need to think critically when informing the doctor of your assessment of the situation. This means that you must consider carefully what might be the underlying reason for your patient's condition. Not only will you have reviewed your findings from your assessment, you will also have consolidated these with other objective indicators, such as laboratory results.

R Recommendation

- Explain what you need – be specific about request and timeframe.
- Make suggestions.
- Clarify expectations.

What is your recommendation? That is, what would you like to happen by the end of the conversation with your colleague?

R Readback

Finally, any order that is given on the phone needs to be repeated back to ensure accuracy.

(www.institute.nhs.uk/quality_and_service_improvement_tools/quality_
and_service_improvement_tools/sbar_-_situation_-_background_-
assessment_-_recommendation.html)

More information about SBARR and its use can be found in Chapter 6.

When should you use SBARR?

SBARR can be used throughout your clinical career in a variety of situations for both urgent and non-urgent communication, when discussing patients with other healthcare professionals, including peers, at handover, and when escalating concerns with seniors. It provides a structure to communication that ensures the most important pieces of information are transmitted in a predictable manner.

ACTIVITY 2.4

Consider the different environments you have been in when you have needed to impart clinical information. Did you use SBARR? What other systems were in place? Did you use a system at all? How did you know that all the information had been imparted correctly and efficiently?

Have you observed SBARR in action? Find out how SBARR is used, if at all, in your most recent placement organisation.

Now look up the NHS Training and Action for Patient Safety (TAPS) website (**www. nhstaps.org/resources/tools**). Listed here are a selection of resources that will provide you with tools to enable safe practice. With a peer, discuss how and when these tools would help improve your practice and therefore help to prevent patient safety incidents.

Communication about patients does not take place solely at the level of the individual and between colleagues on a one-to-one basis. The management of patients and patient safety incidents are also routinely discussed at hospital clinical governance meetings. Each department will have regular clinical governance meetings (perhaps monthly or quarterly). Generally, all members of the healthcare team are expected to attend these meetings and contribute to them by presenting cases, audits or research. Clinical governance meetings are good examples of multidisciplinary and interprofessional work as they bring together people involved in different aspects of patient care. These meetings also often provide an opportunity for trust-wide safety incidents, particularly serious untoward incidents, to be discussed and learned from, within individual departments.

ACTIVITY 2.5 REFLECTION

On your next clinical placement, ask if you can attend a clinical governance meeting. Afterwards, reflect on the following questions.

- How was patient safety discussed at the meeting?
- Did anyone discuss any specific cases or was the conversation more general?
- Was there any assumed knowledge about what is or is not a patient safety incident?
- Whose responsibility is patient safety?
- Who takes the lead in discussions about patient safety?
- Is everyone's opinion sought?

DEFINITION

Clinical governance is defined by the Department of Health (1998, p33) as *a system through which NHS organisations are accountable for continuously improving the quality of their services and safeguarding high standards of care by creating an environment in which excellence in clinical care will flourish.*

The hierarchical structure of healthcare can result in challenges to good communication between professionals regarding patient safety, for example between nurses and doctors and junior and senior clinicians. This hierarchy can also lead to the assumption of the paternalistic model of medicine which assumes that the doctor or healthcare professional 'knows best'. The last decade has witnessed the development of increasing patient and public involvement in healthcare, for example in the White Paper *Equity and Excellence: Liberating the NHS* (Department of Health, 2010a) where the focus is on shared decision-making between patients and clinicians. For further discussion of the benefits and challenges of this approach, see Chapter 3.

Learning point

You are now aware of the informal contexts in which patient safety learning takes place and the importance of communication skills and challenging authority for patient safety.

Innovations in patient safety teaching

Tomorrow's Doctors (General Medical Council, 2009a) and *The Trainee Doctor* (General Medical Council, 2011) both require you to place the patient at the centre of your duties as a doctor. The Royal College of General Practitioners goes further and demands *a new culture that requires a deeper understanding and respect for the patient's agenda coupled with the communication skills, team working and self-awareness to put patient safety into practice* (RCGP Curriculum Statement 3.2: **www.rcgp-curriculum. org.uk/PDF/curr_3_2_Patient_safety.pdf**). How, then, can we facilitate a deeper understanding and respect for the patient's agenda? A systematic review of educational interventions on training on patient safety (Wong *et al.*, 2010) identified a number of programmes integrated into existing undergraduate and/or postgraduate curricula. A number of these were reported as having a positive impact in terms of learner satisfaction and improvements in knowledge and processes of care among the participants. However, the majority of these interventions viewed patient safety with a health professional lens, with a focus on areas such as root cause analysis and patient safety culture. There was relatively limited emphasis on the impact of safety lapses on patients and their families and little or no involvement of patients in the design or delivery of the training.

DEFINITION

Root cause analysis is a problem-solving approach to identifying the cause of a negative outcome or adverse event in a systematic manner. Once the ultimate cause has been established, it becomes possible to plan a way of countering it.

Researchers have attempted to address this issue by engaging the patient as a teacher of patient safety (Jha *et al.*, 2009). This approach allows us to respect patients' agenda by directly involving them, to value the learning opportunities they bring to the patient safety arena and to recognise that ignoring these issues only increases the risk of harm.

What can we learn from the patient about patient safety? Patient narratives

An innovative method of involving patients in education and training of patient safety is the use of patient narratives of harm in a classroom setting (Winterbottom *et al.*, 2010). The narration of a patient safety incident in this manner allows us to come face to face with real-life medical errors and to understand how patients view what has happened to them or their family members. It can help us understand the points at which different choices about care may have taken place, how patients are key resources for understanding the process of doctor–patient communication and how often, in the case of chronic conditions, they are experts in their own care. Listening to patients in this way, with the opportunity to ask questions of patients and discuss the case with peers, offers an opportunity to understand the complex issues and situations that surround most experiences of patient harm. It also allows us to conceive patient safety holistically in the sense that it is not merely an issue for medical professionals but is at the core of your relationship with patients. The format of a textbook does not allow us to recreate the experience of real-life patients narrating their experience of harm. However, reading their stories can help us to understand the importance of patients' perspective in preventing future harm both in terms of their knowledge of themselves and their loved ones and their ability to detect poor practice, for example lack of hand-washing on a particular ward (Weingart *et al.*, 2005; Weissman *et al.*, 2008; King *et al.*, 2010).

Case Study

The following narrative is a real-life example of harm caused to a patient. These events took place in a UK district general hospital. Consider and describe your thoughts and feelings as you read the narrative.

Missed opportunities

My daughter became ill in January 2003. Glandular fever was the suspected illness. She became very poorly with it, requiring hospitalisation. A 24-hour stay in hospital occurred, at which time the medical team showed concern and compassion for how poorly she felt. However, on the basis of it being viral and more a matter of management rather than active treatment, she was sent home. Her condition deteriorated significantly over the next three-day period to the extent that not only was she in much pain, she was completely debilitated and could do nothing for herself. I felt no one really understood how ill she really was.

Following bruise-like markings on her skin both I and her GP suspected meningitis. She was admitted to hospital as an emergency. No tests for meningitis were done but it was concluded that it was not that. She was put on antibiotics as she was so poorly with suspected glandular fever. However, on seeing the same senior medics that had assessed her on her first admission, we were met with an almost annoyed manner that this girl had been sent back in when she had already been assessed and sent home. There was also an annoyance that she had been put on antibiotics for nothing more than glandular fever and was immediately taken off them. She was told she had to simply ride the storm, although they concluded that she could stay in hospital.

Over the next week Louise's condition was worsening every day and I felt very concerned and baffled that no one seemed concerned by anything. Blood tests were being done, so I concluded that should anything show up they would not hesitate to react, especially as they could not treat the glandular fever as such, they surely would treat any complications that should arise from her condition. I felt unheard and that Louise was being dismissed and judged as a 'drama queen' and I was classed as an overprotective mother. Louise herself felt that there was something wrong with her 'pathetic body' as everyone kept telling her she was getting better and she felt she wasn't.

Following many concerned calls to the medical team as well as their normal visits, after seven days on the ward, Louise suffered a massive fit, cardiac arrest, multiorgan failure and DIC [disseminated intravascular coagulation]. On admission to intensive care they diagnosed bacterial toxic shock syndrome and they told me she was a **very** ill young girl: a statement that I had felt to be true for over a week but no one else shared my concern. Her blood tests showed major deterioration two and a half days prior to her complete collapse with the junior doctors highlighting in her notes the drop in platelets from 199 to 50, signs of liver failure, and possible infection. The senior medical team wrote 'getting better'. The following day the haematologist advised further investigation but was overridden by the paediatric consultant and it was written in her records that she was 'feeling better' and her IV drip was withdrawn. On the morning of her collapse her bloods had deteriorated. Her potassium was 6.9 and platelets now 25. She entered ITU [intensive therapy unit] on only oral analgesia administered by me. Two hours after seeing the general ward medical team she was on full life support. She remained on this for two weeks but never regained consciousness. She died from a fungal infection contracted after 11 days on ITU. The postmortem stated that she had brain damage. My feelings at that time and for the rest of my life will be that glandular fever may have always killed Louise but any chance there was to save her and assist her to try and fight this illness and all its complications was missed and that she died in pain with no attempts to try to save her made.

ACTIVITY 2.6

Read slowly through the case study above. What do you think are the main patient safety issues highlighted here?

If you were the junior doctor/health professional in this case, what might you have done differently?

What do you think are some of the advantages/disadvantages of the patient telling the story of these events directly to you?

Possible answer

Some of the main patient safety issues highlighted here are:

- a lack of communication between the medical team, the nursing staff and the patient's family;
- the difficulties associated with team working;
- the challenges of speaking up to seniors.

If you were the junior doctor or health professional in this case, you might have thought about seeking the support of the haematologist to corroborate your concerns and challenge the paediatric consultant.

There are advantages and disadvantages of learning from patients. One advantage is that a first-hand account of a patient safety incident derived directly from the patient or family member offers the opportunity to discuss what went wrong and for the healthcare professional to observe the impact on patients' and professionals' lives. Patients and health professionals have the opportunity to ask questions of one another, which can assist in learning about the causes and consequences of adverse events.

There are some possible disadvantages: health professionals may feel inhibited by the emotional content of the patient's story. This may have a twofold effect: firstly, a desire not to cause further distress to the patient or her family through questioning and secondly, it may trigger upsetting feelings relating to their own experiences, both personal and professional.

This real-life case study brings to the forefront some challenges that exist when working with senior or more experienced colleagues. There are obvious disparities in how Louise appeared to her family and to the senior team. Despite her mother's concerns that she was very unwell, and the fact that the junior members of the team documented the gravity of her illness in her medical records, the senior team did not take these facts on board.

Although challenging more experienced team members about their decision-making can be difficult, it is important for you to remember that it is part of your duty as a doctor to maintain and promote patient safety at all times. Perhaps the junior doctors in this case could have employed more assertive challenges to their seniors? Perhaps they could have approached a senior colleague in another specialty for advice.

It is important to remember that patients and their families are an important source of information about their own condition. In the case above, Louise's mother recognises how unwell her daughter is because of how different her behaviour and general demeanour are compared to her normal state. Information like this is an important component of ensuring safe practice and should be considered alongside the clinical information. It is important for practitioners to remember the context of patients' lives and how this might relate to their presenting condition and therefore to patient safety.

Learning point

You are now able to understand the ways in which we can learn about patient safety from patients themselves and how to work with patients, understanding them as a resource to help you improve patient safety awareness.

What can our colleagues teach us about patient safety?

A recent study conducted by the General Medical Council found that understanding the roles and responsibilities of other healthcare professionals is central to improving patient safety and preventing error. The study reported that *the intervention of nurses, senior doctors and, in particular, pharmacists was vital in picking up errors before they had an impact on patients* (Dornan *et al.*, 2009). Bearing this in mind, it is worth considering how much you understand the roles of your colleagues (for example, nurses, physio-therapists, pharmacists) and what kinds of information they might be able to share that can help to prevent or flag up potential adverse events. This is not about relying on other people to check that you have not made a mistake but rather about working collegially and drawing on the expertise and experience of others in the healthcare team.

One way of understanding the role of other professional groups is to engage in multiprofessional training. Until recently, opportunities for this kind of training have been limited. However, following the House of Commons Health Committee (2009) report on patient safety, which concluded that *those who work together should train together*, more opportunities for such training are emerging. One example is at the University of Leeds, where a pilot project has been carried out to implement an interprofessional training programme on safe prescribing. The teaching session, which is co-facilitated by a medical consultant and a pharmacist, aims to bring together final-year undergraduate students of medicine, pharmacy, dentistry, nursing and midwifery to learn together about safe prescribing. The focus of the teaching is on the elements of safe prescribing, including knowledge of pharmacology, appreciating the role of various health professionals in ensuring safe prescribing practices, communicating with colleagues in case of doubt and the effective use of prescribing guidelines. Using vignettes from real-life examples derived from prior research, these areas are explored in interprofessional groups. There is also a session during which the students get an opportunity to take a detailed, complex drug history from a patient and then write up the prescription. This pilot work has been well received, with students reporting that they are more able to understand the importance of each other's roles within the prescribing team and the help and support that each profession brings to aid safe prescribing safely.

This real-life example demonstrates how a small error can quickly escalate. Firstly, it demonstrates how important it is to check a patient's identity. This is

Case Study: Interprofessional education workshops: prescribing

A locum GP is working in a busy GP-led specialist clinic for asylum seekers in a community centre. The locum GP calls out the patient's name for the 10.30 appointment slot and the patient enters the room.

He prescribes the patient a repeat prescription of medication for depression, fluvoxamine 100mg daily. About 20 minutes later, a nurse practitioner sees the patient who was waiting for the 10.30 appointment in the waiting room. She realises the doctor has prescribed the medication for the wrong patient, who has now left the surgery.

- What do you think happened?
- What would you do next?

The nurse practitioner contacts the local pharmacy which is attached to the community centre, requesting that they do not give out the medication. However, the pharmacist has already given the medication to the patient. She did not check the patient's name or address as he could not speak any English.

- What do you think should be done in this situation?
- How could the pharmacist have checked the patient's details?

When the GP and nurse checked the patient's records they realised he was already taking theophyl line for his asthma, which is dangerous if taken with the antidepressant medication prescription. Fortunately, as the clinic is attached to a community centre, they were able to contact the patient to correct the error.

- Why did this error occur and what could be done to prevent it happening again?

always important, but when communicating with those whose first language is not English extra care must be taken. When prescribing medicines under a repeat prescription it is important to discuss with patients their understanding of the condition being treated and to establish whether repeat prescription is appropriate. In this case, discussion would have highlighted that a repeat prescription for antidepressants was inappropriate. For non-English speakers, using the appropriate translation telephone line may be necessary.

At the pharmacy, care should be taken to check a patient's identity using both name and address to cross-check. Assumptions should not be made that the person who brings in the prescription is the patient.

The case study above is taken from a real-life incident and demonstrates various failures of communication by the team. You can see how easy it is for individual minor oversights suddenly to escalate and lead to more serious incidents. The doctor did not check the patient's identity, nor did he acknowledge his role as a locum with limited patient knowledge or check any details with the nurse practitioner. The pharmacist allowed the language competency of the patient to influence her practice and she also failed to make adequate checks on the patient's identity.

It is important to consider how you will fit into the wider team that works along-side patients, all members of which have a role in maintaining patient safety. At various stages in your career you will interact with others from different professions, all of whom have specialist knowledge, not necessarily clinical in nature, but that can promote safe practice.

Good working communication between members of the team, perhaps from those who know the patient or patient group well (e.g. in the case of the nurse prac-titioner and the locum GP) is essential. Language barriers are common in medical practice but effort is required to double-check that the correct patient is present in the surgery. In this case, if the locum GP was unsure about patient identity, he should have checked with another member of the team. In this way, he would have drawn upon and acknowledged the specialist patient knowledge that existed within the team.

Learning point

You are now able to recognise how learning from and with other healthcare profes-sionals, not necessarily your seniors, is vital to improving your knowledge about patient safety.

How can you ensure patient safety remains a key focus throughout your career?

Due to rapid developments in all aspects of medicine, including investigations, therapeutics and management, it is sometimes quite a challenge to keep pace with the changes. If all doctors simply relied on knowledge gained during medical school or postgraduate education, we would all rapidly become outdated in our knowledge and skills and this would have a major impact on patient safety. The evidence base for what constitutes safe practice changes with new research findings; these changes are reflected in new guidelines from national organisations such as the National Institute for Health and Clinical Excellence or the Royal Colleges. It is now manda-tory for all doctors to engage in continuing professional development to keep their practice safe and up to date. This is an integral part of revalidation plans from the General Medical Council that will require doctors to demonstrate continuing learn-ing and skills development throughout their career.

> Unequivocally, revalidation is our top priority. This is what we believe is the most important thing in advancing the quality of medical regulation and having an impact in the long term in improving patient safety.
>
> (Niall Dickson, General Medical Council, 28 October 2010)

You have now learned how keeping up to date with developments in research and continuing professional development is a vital component for ensuring safe practice throughout your medical career.

Chapter summary

Patient safety is an essential component of professional guidelines and therefore key to your future career as a doctor. This chapter has looked at some of the contexts in which you can learn about patient safety, for example in your undergraduate curriculum, on clinical placements, from other colleagues and from patients themselves. It has provided you with useful tools for improving your communication skills, including PACE and SBARR, and has stressed the importance of continuing professional development in ensuring safe practice.

Patient safety is best approached in a holistic manner which allows team members to challenge appropriately, draw on each other's experience and expertise and put patients at the centre of their care in a way that fosters safe practice. It is not always easy to prevent errors but, by acknowledging the complexities of medical practice, and by recognising and appreciating how and why errors might occur, you will be better placed to draw on the resources available to you to promote patient safety.

What you have learned in this chapter:

- why patient safety is integral to the General Medical Council and other regulatory bodies, for example the Royal Colleges' guidelines;
- how learning about patient safety is holistic and takes place in formal and informal settings;
- patient-led innovations in teaching about patient safety, such as using patient narratives (or narratives by relatives of patients) for case studies;
- how interprofessional co-operation can increase your ability to practise safely as a doctor;
- why continuing professional development is central to continuing to practise safely throughout your career.

GOING FURTHER

To read more about practising safely as a trainee, have a look at How to be Safer Doctors: A guide for doctors in training at: **www.institute.nhs.uk/images// documents/SaferCare/Library/A5%20How%20to%20be%20safer% 20doctors-AW.pdf**.

Use online sources to help you develop your skills and knowledge in patient safety education: **www.nhstaps.org**.

Read more about the background to the implementation of SBARR in the NHS: **www.institute.nhs.uk/quality_and_service_improvement_tools/ quality_and_service_improvement_tools/sbar_-_situation_-_ background_-_assessment_-_recommendation.html**.

Discover tutorials to help you learn about situational awareness and how this might influence your practice and patient safety: **www.training-pod.com/savi/**.

Read more about prescribing errors in Dornan's work: **www.gmc-uk.org/about/research/research_commissioned_4.asp**.

Why revalidation (so lifelong learning as a practitioner) enhances patient safety: **www.gmc-uk.org/news/8133.asp**.

Listen to the General Medical Council's revalidation podcast: **www.gmc-uk.org/doctors/revalidation/podcast_4.asp**.

Acknowledgements

We would like to thank Carolyn Cleveland for her permission to include the story of her daughter's experience in this chapter. We also thank Helen Bradbury for her help in preparing the prescribing case study.

chapter 3

Involving Patients in Their Own Safety

*Jane Ward, Sally Giles,
Susan Hrisos, Penny Rhodes,
Ikhlaq Din and Peter Walsh*

Achieving your medical degree

This chapter will help you to meet the following requirements of *Tomorrow's Doctors* (General Medical Council, 2009a).

Outcome 2: The doctor as a practitioner

The graduate will be able to:

13. Carry out a consultation with a patient:

   (b) Elicit patients' questions, their understanding of their condition and treatment options, and their views, concerns, values and preferences.
   (f) Determine the extent to which patients want to be involved in decision-making about their care and treatment.
   (g) Provide explanation, advice, reassurance and support.

14. Diagnose and manage clinical presentations:

   (c) Formulate a plan of investigation in partnership with the patient, obtaining informed consent as an essential part of this process.
   (g) Formulate a plan for treatment, management and discharge, according to established principles and best evidence, in partnership with patients, their carers, and other health professionals as appropriate. Respond to patients' concerns and preferences, obtain informed consent, and respect the rights of patients to reach decisions with their doctor about their treatment and care and to refuse or limit treatment.

15. Communicate effectively with patients and colleagues in a medical context:

   (b) Communicate clearly, sensitively and effectively with individuals and groups regardless of their age, social, cultural or ethnic backgrounds or their disabilities, including when English is not the patient's first language.

Outcome 3: The doctor as a professional

The graduate will be able to:

20. Behave according to ethical and legal principles:

    (b) Demonstrate awareness of the clinical responsibilities and role of the doctor, making the care of the patient the first concern. Recognise the principles of patient-centred care, including self-care, and deal with patients' healthcare needs in consultation with them and, where appropriate, their relatives or carers.

Chapter overview

By definition, there are no health professionals without patients. The delivery of care is embedded within a partnership, with patients, their relatives and carers and health professionals each playing their role to help ensure a positive outcome for the patient. This partnership also applies to patient safety, and it is important for medical practitioners to understand and appreciate the role of patients in helping to promote the safety of themselves and others, while receiving treatment within a healthcare setting.

In this chapter we present some ways in which patients and their relatives and carers can be involved in the safety of their care. We discuss current initiatives and new innovations that aim to provide a platform for patient involvement, and the benefits and challenges of such involvement. We consider the factors that may influence the degree to which any given patient might be willing and able to be involved in his or her own safety. Finally, we will help you identify steps you can take to facilitate and encourage patient involvement within your practice.

After reading this chapter you will be able to:

- explore when and how patients can be involved in their own safety;
- understand the potential benefits and challenges of patient involvement;
- discuss whether patient involvement is appropriate or beneficial for all patients all of the time;
- have some ideas about what you, as a health professional, can do to encourage such involvement.

Introduction

The safety of patients has traditionally been viewed as the concern of health professionals, with patients themselves seen as passive recipients of healthcare. More recently, this view has shifted slightly, with the patient voice emerging as a key part of healthcare provision within the UK and internationally. A key driver for this shift in focus was the recent political move towards patient choice as part of creating a more dynamic and responsive health service. This change in policy was aimed at empowering patients to be active partners in their own healthcare. Indeed, within the UK, the government is clear that for NHS patients there should be *no decision about me, without me* (Department of Health, 2010b).

One way in which patients can act as partners in their care is to be involved in the process of monitoring (and at times, help manage) the safety of both themselves and others in healthcare settings. At a policy level within the UK this has been highlighted in a number of government reports, publications and White Papers (Department of Health, 2004, 2008, 2010). The move to involve patients in patient safety has also been driven by patients, their families and patient organisations. For example, the charity Action against Medical Accidents has championed the cause of patient involvement in patient safety in the UK, and managed the Patients for Patient Safety project, initially in partnership with the National Patient Safety Agency (NPSA), and now independently. The Patients for Patient Safety project has also been extended internationally, as a work stream of the World Health Organization. In line with this change in perspective, around a decade ago researchers began to consider how patients, their relatives and carers might be involved in patient safety initiatives. The emerging consensus from this small, but steadily growing, body of work is that patients can be meaningfully involved in their own safety in a range of healthcare settings.

So, it is clear that patient involvement is now an important part of healthcare delivery, and is likely to remain so for the foreseeable future. But what does this actually mean for healthcare professionals?

When and how can patients be involved in their safety?

This first section focuses on the different ways that patients are currently asked to be involved in their safety, as well as the innovations in patient involvement.

Current initiatives

Promoting safety and preventing adverse events

There are several different approaches to encouraging patients to get involved in promoting safer health care. One approach is national campaigning, which aims to encourage patients to take a more informed and proactive role in their healthcare. An example of this from the USA is the Joint Commission initiative Speak Up, which has a general focus on helping patients to be involved in preventing medical error. Patients are encouraged to be vigilant about the care they receive, to ask questions and to voice any concerns they may have. Other initiatives address specific aspects of care, an example being the Clean your Hands campaign, initiated in the UK by the NPSA, to encourage patients to ask health professionals if they have washed their hands. However, the success of such campaigns has yet to be fully established. Indeed, although Clean your Hands was associated with a reduction in infections, its success in terms of encouraging patients to challenge healthcare professionals was limited (Stone *et al.*, 2007).

More successful, perhaps, are initiatives that focus on patients with long-term conditions, who are more likely to develop lasting relationships with health professionals. Patients who have ongoing treatment may be better placed to identify errors or lapses, as they become more knowledgeable and familiar with the details of their care, than those experiencing single episodes of care (Weingart *et al.*, 2007). Successful examples include initiatives to involve patients undergoing repeated episodes of chemotherapy and renal dialysis patients (Schwappach and Wernli, 2010; **www. renalpatientview.org/index.do**).

Preventing and ameliorating harm following a patient safety incident

Another way that patients can be involved in their safety is by helping to prevent harm, or ameliorate further harm once a patient safety incident (PSI) has occurred. A PSI is defined by the NPSA as *any unintended or unexpected incident which could have or did lead to harm for one or more patients receiving NHS care*. Currently, patients are routinely asked to identify adverse drug reactions (ADRs), and the literature suggests that patients make a valuable contribution in this regard (Egberts *et al.*, 1996; Blenkinsopp *et al.*, 2006). Indeed, there are a number of advantages of patients reporting ADRs: patients are often able to respond more quickly than healthcare professionals (Egberts *et al.*, 1996), and the types of ADRs patients report differ from those identified by health professionals, particularly for new drugs (van den Bemt *et al.*, 1999). Patient reporting may also contribute to the earlier detection of ADRs (Egberts *et al.*, 1996).

Innovations

Patient incident reporting

Within the UK, at a national level the NPSA invites patients to report any safety 'experiences' they have had through the National Reporting and Learning System.

ACTIVITY 3.1

Have a look at the NPSA National Reporting and Learning System website: **www. nrls.npsa.nhs.uk/**.

As you will see, all published reports only deal with incident reports from health professionals. There are no published reports concerning patient-reported data. In a small group, discuss why you think they may have little patient-reported data?

At a local level, current systems for collecting patient reports about safety concerns generally focus on complaints processes. Whilst these do provide healthcare organisations with vital information about how to manage safety better in the future, they are limited in their scope, usually dealing with more serious safety concerns for patients. Furthermore, in dealing with complaints, healthcare organisations may not actually involve patients at all, resulting in lost opportunities for individual and organisational learning.

To date, patients have rarely been asked to report routinely on safety problems experienced during their care, using formal incident reporting systems. However, growing evidence from the literature indicates that patients are not only in a position to report PSIs, but are also willing to do so (King *et al.*, 2010; Schwappach, 2010). In research studies at least, it seems that when routinely asked to report on their safety in hospital, patients provide a wide range of experiences, from service quality events through to the more severe and life-threatening PSIs (Weingart *et al.*, 2005).

This variety of PSIs reported by patients presents healthcare organisations with the possibility of learning not only retrospectively from more serious events, but also prospectively from data about minor PSIs. This approach is currently being trialled in a large-scale UK-based study which aims to develop a patient-led patient incident reporting system, to allow healthcare organisations to capture routinely safety concerns from patients (as well as relatives or carers) while staying in hospital (Ward *et al.*, 2011). It is hoped that such a system will go some way towards filling the current gap between patients experiencing safety concerns and making a formal complaint.

Patients reporting on the safety of the clinical environment

Patients are also able to comment on more general safety issues which extend beyond their own care and include the ward, hospital or clinical environment and the care of other patients (Weingart *et al.*, 2007). In addition, from the patient vista they may well be in a position to identify issues that healthcare professionals do not always recognise or may not be in a position to observe (Davis *et al.*, 2008). For example, patients might be better placed than health professionals to observe another patient about to fall out of bed or suddenly deteriorate, the care of more vulnerable patients (e.g. chronically ill patients, or perhaps those who do not speak English), as well as lapses in infection control behaviours. In recognition of the potential role of patients in reporting on safety climate, there is currently work underway to develop a Patient Measure of Organisational Safety (Ward *et al.*, 2011). It is anticipated that such a measure will help to elicit the views of patients (and their relatives or carers) about the care environment. It may even be possible to use this as a leading patient safety indicator to enable healthcare organisations to manage patient safety proactively.

ACTIVITY 3.2   EXAMPLE OF A PATIENT SAFETY INCIDENT FROM A PATIENT'S PERSPECTIVE

Setting: A cardiology ward in a large teaching hospital

An 80-year-old female patient was admitted to the cardiology ward following a myocardial infarction. The patient was given appropriate treatment and was on the road to recovery. On this ward, it had previously been recognised that staff did not engage enough with patients, so they had recently introduced a new initiative where a senior nurse would spend a few minutes each day asking patients how they were, and if they had any problems. About a week after the patient had been admitted, she was approached in the morning by the ward sister who asked how she was, to which she replied, 'I am fine'. Despite saying to the nurse that she was fine, the patient had been experiencing chest pain all morning. She could see the staff were busy and didn't want to bother them with something she thought might be perceived as too trivial, or be labelled as a trouble-maker. On a previous occasion the patient had seen a fellow patient being addressed in a 'short' manner by a nurse, which made her reluctant to raise her own concerns. The patient's condition deteriorated and she suffered another myocardial infarction. Fortunately, she was given the necessary treatment and survived this episode.

1. *In a small group think about what happened. Each of you should consider the case study and write a couple of sentences describing how you respond to the situation described. Share your responses.*

   This is a clear example of a PSI that could have been prevented. In spite of an initiative on this ward to encourage interaction between patients and ward staff, this PSI still happened. Communication between the nurse and patient took place, but it was not effective in terms of uncovering the information that would have highlighted the problems the patient was experiencing.

2. *In your small group, discuss what you think the role of the patient was.*

   In this case, the patient was fully aware that she was experiencing chest pain. It was her role to mention this to a member of staff and she was given the opportunity to do this when the nurse asked her how she was. Despite this, the patient felt unable to raise her concerns with the nurse, as she did not want to bother nurses, who gave the impression of being too busy to spend time talking. She was afraid of being labelled as a 'moaner' or receiving a response similar to that she had witnessed with another patient.

3. *Individually, list three ways in which you think that communication between staff and patients might be improved on this ward. Then share your three ways with others in your small group. Are you surprised by the overlap (or lack of overlap) in the points raised?*

   Despite the provision of an initiative to encourage interaction between staff and patients and to give patients the opportunity to voice their concerns, this patient still felt unable to tell the staff about her chest pain. It shows that patient involvement is not just a 'tick box' exercise and that some thought needs to go into the process of ongoing communication with patients where trusting relationships are formed, so they feel comfortable to voice their concerns. There is also the danger with an initiative like this one that other members of staff believe that patients have already been asked how they are, so do not feel the need to ask them again. This is a clear example of an initiative that was implemented to encourage patients to speak up but, because of the way it was managed and not embedded in everyone's responsibility, resulted in a PSI.

This section has considered current and future initiatives aimed at involving patients in their safety within a healthcare setting. It is clear that there are a variety of ways in which patients may become involved in safety-related behaviours, although due to the emerging nature of research in this area, more work needs to be done to understand the full impact of such involvement on the wider patient safety performance of a healthcare organisation. There is, however, a growing understanding of how patient involvement may impact upon individual patients and health professionals. The next section considers the evidence for both the benefits and challenges of involving patients in their safety.

What are the potential benefits and challenges of patient involvement?

Benefits of patient involvement

Most experts in the field believe that patients have a place in making their care safer (Donabedian, 1992; Entwistle, 2007; Donaldson, 2008; Leape *et al.*, 2009) and evidence suggests that many patients are not only willing and able to participate in improving their safety and improving health outcomes, but that such a role also has the potential to improve safety (Donaldson, 2008; Pronovost *et al.*, 2009).

Patients as your partners in their care

Patients and their families have a unique perspective on their experience of healthcare and can provide information and insights that healthcare professionals may not otherwise have known (Donaldson, 2008). With this in mind, viewing them as partners in their care could greatly enhance the safety of your clinical practice (Entwistle, 2007). For example, taking time to listen to what patients say about their symptoms or concerns could help you in reaching a more accurate diagnosis or to identify deterioration or side effects of medications more promptly (Vincent and Coulter, 2002). Taking time to explain aspects of their care to patients also has benefits. Lowe and colleagues (2000) provided older people with tailored education about their medicines as part of a medicine review programme. They found that this led to an increase in patients' understanding of the purpose of their medicines and improved compliance with their medication regimes. Similarly, involving patients in decisions about their treatment has been demonstrated to improve concordance with, and adherence to, agreed treatment regimens (Joosten *et al.*, 2008).

An extra barrier to harm

Patients (and in some situations, their relatives too) can act as an 'extra barrier' or 'safety buffer' against avoidable harm (Johnstone and Kanistaki, 2009). Again, involving patients and their families by talking to and educating them about the patient's care puts them in a better position to help avoid adverse events happening (Longtin *et al.*, 2010), especially if they are told in advance about what to expect (Entwistle, 2007). For example, patients could partner with healthcare professionals as a final check on the accuracy of any medications they are given, or to verify the correct surgical site prior to going to theatre. Thinking about medications administration, such partnering might simply involve communicating with patients, in a conversational way, what drugs you are about to administer and why, and asking them if this is what they are expecting to receive (Entwistle, 2007). Such collaborative actions not only offer enhanced safety and an opportunity for you to provide education, but also demonstrate your respect for that patient as a person. This can also serve to reassure patients about their safety and care, while engendering trust in caregivers (Entwistle, 2007).

Another piece in the error detection 'jigsaw'

There is growing evidence that no single error detection method (e.g. staff incident reporting, case note review, complaints) provides the full picture of PSIs across a healthcare organisation, with different methods only overlapping slightly in terms of the PSIs identified (Franklin *et al.*, 2009; Naessens *et al.*, 2009). It is clear that patient involvement, particularly in highlighting safety concerns, may offer healthcare organisations another means of learning about safety, in order to manage it better in the future. There is early evidence of this from a 2010 study in which patients were found to report very different medication problems from those identified through medical or nursing staff reporting, or through traditional case note review (Kaboli *et al.*, 2010). In this study, while patients reported in similar numbers to nurses and physicians, they reported more adverse drug events than medical error when com-pared with health professional reports.

Challenges of patient involvement

While we can see that there are mutually valuable benefits to be gained from involv-ing patients and their families in efforts to maintain high standards of safety, some potential challenges of such participation exist.

Erosion of trust

Concerns have been expressed by some authors that raising patient awareness of safety issues will undermine patients' notion of safety within healthcare settings and possibly even deter some patients from seeking care (Lyons, 2007). Approaches to promoting patient involvement that prompt patients to 'challenge' healthcare pro-fessionals (for example, 'ask your healthcare professional if they have washed their hands') are seen as having a particular potential for damaging the patient–practitioner relationship (Entwistle *et al.*, 2005). It is also important to remember that patients can be hesitant in raising with health professionals concerns that they may consider to be too trivial, as they are often able to see how overworked and busy they can be (Entwistle *et al.*, 2010). In addition, patients may fear the repercussions of reporting. For example, they may fear being rebuffed by healthcare professionals, or that their care may somehow be compromised if they speak up, especially if they are relatively dependent on professional help (Entwistle *et al.*, 2010).

Vulnerability of patients

Patients across a variety of care settings are likely at some stage to feel vulnerable, due to the need to place their trust in health professionals. It is possible that increased patient involvement might risk inappropriately shifting responsibility for safety onto already vulnerable patients (Entwistle *et al.*, 2005). Some have argued that an over-reliance on patients could also inadvertently lull healthcare professionals into a false sense of safety (Lyons, 2007) and risks creating inequalities between those patients who do, and those who do not, actively engage in their healthcare (Johnstone and Kanistaki, 2009). Furthermore, we need to be mindful that a more realistic evaluation of risk may engender greater anxiety in patients. The responsibility for patients' safety must therefore remain with healthcare professionals, but with a partnership approach where patient involvement is encouraged, although never assumed.

ACTIVITY 3.3

Imagine you have been asked to introduce a patient involvement initiative in your clinical area. This initiative invites patients to ask health professionals if they have washed their hands before any patient contact. How would you go about discussing the benefits and challenges of this particular intervention with firstly, your clinical colleagues, and secondly, patients and their families?

Points to consider:

1. **Clinical colleagues**
   Include in the introduction a discussion about the rationale for this approach and why it has been suggested as a useful approach to enhancing patient safety, e.g.:

- Health professionals sometimes forget, so it is a helpful prompt if patients or relatives ask.
- It may help to maintain high standards as a safe practitioner.
- Patients are concerned about infection so hand-washing reassures them.
- It reduces the risk of cross-contamination between patients.
- Challenges may include time constraints, and the 'challenging' nature of such an approach to the health professional.

2. **Patients and their families**
   Try to speak to individual patients about this initiative, as this may encourage their involvement.

- Stress that asking does not mean 'challenging'.
- Try to create a permissive atmosphere between health professionals and patients.
- Emphasise how the initiative helps health professionals maintain high standards of care.

This section has highlighted just some of the potential benefits – and pitfalls – in involving patients in their own safety. You will probably be able to think of other issues that may arise when asking patients to be partners in their care. The important point from all of the above is that, while the benefits are potentially great for patients, health professionals and healthcare organisations, there are also challenges. Thought must therefore be given in each individual patient interaction about the needs of the patient (and, where appropriate, relatives or carers) and the degree to which involvement is appropriate and timely. We turn to this latter process in the following section.

Is involvement appropriate for all patients, all of the time?

The preceding two sections highlight that, in general, patients are able to participate in their safety, but there are both benefits and challenges to this involvement. Although it is important to understand generally how patients might approach greater involvement in their safety, we also need to consider that patients might vary in the degree to which they are willing and able to get involved.

So, do patients universally want to be involved in their safety? The evidence from clinical decision-making research suggests that some patients may be unwilling to take part in decisions about their care (Longtin *et al.*, 2010). In terms of patient safety, this also seems to apply.

What factors influence patients' ability or willingness to be involved in their safety?

One of the most important issues for health professionals to consider when involving patients in their care and safety is the degree to which patients might be willing – or able – to participate meaningfully in this involvement. So what can research tell us about this? Although this is a relatively new area for patient safety researchers, there is growing evidence about a number of factors which may affect the appropriateness of patient involvement for any given patient.

Age

There is some evidence that older patients are less likely to want to participate in safety-related behaviours (Waterman *et al.*, 2006). Indeed, it is generally acknowledged that older patients are less interested in acting as partners in clinical decision-making (Levinson *et al.*, 2005). However, given that older patients may experience a greater number of adverse events (Sari *et al.*, 2008), and arguably be more likely to have greater illness severity and number of complicating comorbidities, it is important for health professionals to be creative in methods of engagement with this patient group.

Condition and illness severity

Both the nature and severity of the patient's condition may well impact on that patient's ability and desire to be involved in safety-related behaviours. Although this has yet to be established with respect to patient safety, research from decision-making suggests that, for most conditions, patients' desire to be partners in their care decreases as their illness severity increases (Longtin *et al.*, 2010). However, this may be more complicated for patients with chronic conditions, who either receive ongoing treatment or who experience repeat presentations at hospital. It has been suggested that such patients might be in a better position to recognise lapses in their care (Entwistle *et al.*, 2010), and may be more likely to get involved in patient involvement initiatives due to the trust gained in the longer-term relationships built up with staff (Weingart *et al.*, 2007). However, other evidence suggests that those patients receiving ongoing treatment may moderate their behaviour in order to 'do what is right' and 'please the nurse' (Waterworth and Luker, 1990). Given the equivocal evidence, it is perhaps wise for health professionals simply to be mindful that, while patients with chronic illness may be a valuable source of information about their safety, their willingness to engage in patient involvement initiatives may need to be encouraged through a partnership approach.

Ethnicity

Not much is known about the role of ethnicity, culture and language in patients' willingness or ability to be involved in their safety. It is known, however, that patients who have limited proficiency in English, but who are receiving treatment in an English-speaking country, may be more at risk of experiencing a PSI (Divi *et al.*, 2007). Ethnic differences have also been shown with respect to more general patient participation (Cooper-Patrick *et al.*, 1999; Levinson *et al.*, 2005). It may be important, therefore, for health professionals to make efforts to engage creatively with ethnic minority patients in terms of their care. The next section considers creative ways of engaging with patients from different cultures.

Socioeconomic status (SES)

There is evidence to suggest that patients with higher levels of education and patients in paid employment are more likely to ask questions of both medical and nursing staff (Davis *et al.*, 2008). Furthermore, medical staff have been shown to change their communication style on the basis of SES, with lower SES patients experiencing more directive, less participatory interactions (Willems *et al.*, 2005). It may be important therefore for health professionals to understand how patients' SES level may impact on their ability to be involved in their safety, and to ensure an appropriate response based on patient feedback and not on stereotypical beliefs or preconceptions.

Self-efficacy

There is some evidence to suggest that the greater a patient's level of self-efficacy in preventing error, the more likely he or she is to engage in preventive action (Hibbard *et al.*, 2005). It seems that self-efficacy is related to previous experience of hospital, meaning that patients with recent experience may feel more comfortable engaging in safety-related behaviours. Information about preventing error has also been shown to increase patient self-efficacy for preventing error (Hibbard *et al.*, 2005; Schwappach and Wernli, 2010), indicating that basic information may be helpful in encouraging patient engagement.

Healthcare professionals' role or specialty

Whilst there is some evidence to suggest that patients are prepared to ask questions of healthcare professionals, they may be less likely to ask what they perceive to be 'challenging' safety questions (i.e. non-factual) of medical staff compared to nursing staff (Davis *et al.*, 2008, 2011).

The type of patient involvement

The type of involvement may well influence a patient's likelihood of involvement in safety-related behaviours. For example, asking health professionals about issues such as hand-washing or marking surgical sites has been shown to be far more difficult for patients than asking questions about their health or routine care (Waterman *et al.*, 2006; Davis *et al.*, 2011). Indeed, patient involvement initiatives which ask patients to undertake 'non-traditional' actions or roles (e.g. asking challenging questions) seem to be less likely to secure patient engagement (Waterman *et al.*, 2006; Schwappach and Wernli, 2010; Davis *et al.*, 2011).

ACTIVITY 3.4   CASE STUDIES

There follow three separate background descriptions of patients. Please reflect on each in turn, and consider what level of involvement in their safety we might expect for the three patients. Write down your thoughts before turning to the 'points to consider' section below.

Patient A

A 45-year-old male patient with end-stage renal failure has been admitted to your ward with acute peritonitis. He is currently in a great deal of pain and receiving pain-relieving medications, as well as intraperitoneal and intravenous antibiotics. The medical team expect him to make a full recovery from this acute period of illness, and return to routine dialysis regimen.

Patient B

A 32-year-old non-English-speaking female patient is referred to your ward with acute-onset non-specific abdominal pain. She is undergoing a series of tests to identify any underlying pathology, but a diagnosis has not yet been agreed. The duration of her stay in hospital is as yet unknown. She is visited by her husband and teenage daughter daily.

Patient C

An 80-year-old white, male, former senior executive has been admitted to your ward for routine elective cataract surgery. He is likely to stay in overnight following the surgery, and is not expected to experience any complications.

Points to consider

Patient A

This patient is currently experiencing an acute episode of illness, but within the context of a chronic disease. Therefore, although he may currently be unable to participate in safety initiatives, this may change when he has recovered from this acute period of illness. Indeed, due to the chronic nature of his condition, he will most likely be knowledgeable about his care and therefore able to contribute positively in safety initiatives.

Patient B

This patient's non-specific condition may mean that she is subject to a great deal of contact with health professionals during the diagnostic process. Clearly, this contact would need to be facilitated either through interpreters or via her relatives (husband and daughter visiting daily). It is important to remember, however, that there may also be other – culturally bound – barriers to communication. For example, in some cultures a female would need to have a male chaperone when speaking to health professionals (particularly male staff). Additional issues might be that in some cultures (especially non-western cultures), authority is respected and any challenge is discouraged.

Patient C

On the basis that this patient is relatively well, only undergoing routine minor surgery and comes from a professional background, this patient may be more likely to ask direct questions of health professionals, as well as provide information relevant to treatment and safety. However, other factors may need to be considered. For example, this is an older patient who by virtue of his age may be more accustomed to a paternalistic model of care. Therefore, direct questioning of health professionals may be challenging for him. In addition, some elderly patients may not have relatives or friends visiting, reducing the options for engagement with other involved parties.

This section has demonstrated that a number of factors might influence patients' ability or willingness to be more involved in their safety. The list of factors is not exhaustive, and you will be able to think of other factors that might also affect a patient's likelihood of engaging with health professionals in safety matters. As a health professional, the important issue is to be aware of the potential differences in the appropriateness of involvement between patients – as well as the potential differences for the same patient at different points in the treatment trajectory – and to take steps to accommodate these differences into your practice. Furthermore, just because patients may be able to participate, willingness should never be assumed. Ultimately, patients should always be allowed to choose their level of involvement.

What can you do as a health professional to encourage patient involvement?

So far we have identified different ways that patients might get involved in safety-related behaviours, the benefits and challenges of such involvement and the factors that might influence such involvement. This next section deals with what you as a health professional might do to encourage patients to become more involved.

Evidence-based approaches to encouraging patient involvement

Invite patients to engage with you

It has been demonstrated that patients are more likely to want to engage with health professionals, and be prepared to ask questions that might be seen to 'challenge', when invited to do so by health professionals (Davis *et al.*, 2008). Furthermore, patients report that, when health professionals give the impression of caring, having time and welcoming the contributions of patients, they are more likely to speak up about safety concerns (Entwistle *et al.*, 2010). Building a partnership of trust might be an important step for health professionals to gain better engagement from patients.

What's the evidence?

To date, there is little empirical evidence about how to engage practically with patients about patient safety. However, there is evidence from other literatures that suggests that even small changes to practice can help engage patients. John Heritage and colleagues (2006) conducted a study that examined different ways of concluding general practice consultations. They asked physicians to *gaze directly at the patient, and avoid looking at the medical record*, and conclude the consultation with one of two statements:

1. 'Is there *anything* else you want to address in the visit today?'
2. 'Is there *something* else you want to address in the visit today?'

Before the consultation patients were asked to list any concerns they had that they wished to discuss with the physician. All consultations were video-taped, and in analysis, the researchers then identified if the patients had left the consultation with any 'unmet concerns' (i.e. concerns that patients had identified preconsultation, but were not raised by them or addressed by physicians during the consultation).

Which of these two questions do you think was more successful at getting patients to discuss their concerns?

- The first statement, which is widely promoted in textbooks about medical consultations, proved relatively ineffective. No statistically significant difference was found between the control group (i.e. no statement at the end of the visit), and the 'any' statement, in terms of the incidence of patients' 'unmet concerns'.
- Compared with the control group, the second statement strongly reduced the incidence of patients feeling that they left the visit with 'unmet concerns'. More importantly, this effect was achieved without significantly increasing visit length, or generating 'unanticipated' concerns.

Provide information to patients about their care

Limiting the amount of information provided to patients, their relatives and carers can serve to maintain the perceived power imbalance between health professionals and patients (Henderson, 2003). Furthermore, patients receiving conflicting information might be less able to identify safety concerns when they experience them (Entwistle *et al.*, 2010). Indeed, as highlighted in the previous section, providing information to patients about how they might be involved in their safety can help to increase self-efficacy to be involved in safety-related behaviours, which may ultimately lead to increased engagement in such behaviours (Hibbard *et al.*, 2005). It may be important, therefore, for health professionals to provide patients with thorough and consistent information about their care, as well as their role in patient safety, in order to facilitate patient involvement.

Be an honest and open communicator

Failures in communication between health professionals are known to be a key contributory factor in PSIs (Sutcliffe *et al.*, 2004). Given the complexity of the delivery of healthcare, this is perhaps not surprising. However, problems with communication may also be manifested within the health professional–patient relationship. As already discussed, a prerequisite for patients (or relatives and carers) to be involved-proactively in their safety is that information is exchanged between the patient and health professional as part of a constructive dialogue. However, communicating effectively with patients, their relatives and carers is also a vital part of the process of dealing with PSIs after they have happened. Indeed, the NHS Constitution for England (Department of Health, 2010b) states that:

> The NHS also commits when mistakes happen, to acknowledge them, apologise, explain what went wrong and put things right quickly and effectively.

Being open with patients about PSIs that have occurred is important for patients. Patients and families consistently report that they would like disclosure following an incident (Croskerry, 2009a). Indeed, it has been suggested that, even when formal action has been taken by a patient following a PSI, patients primarily want communication, information and apologies from their health professionals rather than litigious retribution or compensation (Walker, 2004). In the spirit of open disclosure, patient charities have recently called for an organisational 'duty of candour' to complement health professionals' personal duty to be open with patients (Action against Medical Accidents, 2011). There may also be benefits in being open following a PSI for health professionals, with the retention of good patient relationships appearing to increase the likelihood of a positive emotional response to the incident for the health professional (Croskerry, 2009b).

ACTIVITY 3.5

The NPSA (2009) Patient Safety Alert: NPSA/2009/PSA003 outlines the actions required by NHS organisations following the revision of the Being Open policy. As part of the guidance, there are some e-learning modules that help illustrate how medical professionals can put the Being Open policy into practice.

Be creative in ways of engaging with patients

One of the central messages of this chapter is that, while we can generalise to a large extent about many issues in patient involvement, consideration must be given to individual patients and their particular circumstances when deciding upon an appropriate level of involvement. To this end, as health professionals you will need to 'individualise' your practice for each patient, encouraging and guiding involvement in different ways, and to varying extents. The very process of individualising your practice – seeing your patient as a 'person' and not a 'case' – may well encourage patient involvement (Entwistle *et al.*, 2010).

You may, however, have to be creative in engaging some patients. This may be relatively straightforward for some patients. For example, with those unable to be involved in safety initiatives due to not speaking the language or perhaps other factors such as acuity, or physical or mental capacity, involvement might be allowed 'by proxy' through involving relatives, carers or even other patients. Indeed, it has been suggested that problems in involving patients where there is a language divide, may to a large extent be ameliorated by language facilitation or the involvement of family members (Garrett *et al.*, 2008). It has also been demonstrated that parents are able to report critical incidents occurring during the care of their children in paediatric intensive care (Frey *et al.*, 2009). It is clear, therefore, that even if patients themselves cannot be involved in their safety, there may be other ways to gain their 'proxy' involvement via other people.

For other patients, however, engagement may be a more complicated process. For patients with a different cultural background to one's own, developing transcultural competence will be important for your practice. It is recognised that there is a need for health professionals to understand the diversity of interpretations of health and illness among cultural groups (Gerrish and Papadopoulos, 1999). For example, the western medical model of healthcare delivery may not always be understood or valued by patients from non-western cultures. In general terms, developing transcultural competence may involve: (1) an understanding of culture and how it shapes identity; (2) knowledge about ethnicity and cultural identity; (3) developing communication skills to facilitate successful cultural encounters; (4) an understanding of health, ill health and healthcare with respect to culture (e.g. preferences for care, strategies for self-care, illness beliefs); and (5) the importance of social and cultural context (e.g. gender dynamics, family pressures/dynamics, religious beliefs) (Jirwe *et al.*, 2009).

ACTIVITY 3.6   SCENARIO

You are a male gynaecologist working the night shift on a surgical ward. You are treating a 25-year-old South Asian female who has a possible ectopic pregnancy. She needs urgent treatment, and you are the senior medical professional on call. What are the issues you should consider in trying to engage with this patient?

- Does she speak English? If not, you will need an interpreter or a family member, although not all patients in this situation would want to use an interpreter who is not a family member.
- Is she on her own? If she is not accompanied by her husband or a family member then you may need to find someone to act as a chaperone. It may be acceptable for this to be a female colleague, but you would need to establish this with the patient first.
- What is the patient's acuity? Your first priority will always be the safety of your patient. When the situation is urgent, you may judge that cultural issues will be superseded by the need to treat the patient in a timely manner, although this may need to be justified after the event.

*Accept the challenge of patient involvement to the traditional authority of
the health professional*

Perhaps one of the most important issues to consider is how you feel about patient
involvement. It is known that a major barrier to general patient participation is
the reluctance of health professionals to acknowledge and embrace the new role
for patients in healthcare delivery (Longtin *et al.*, 2010). For example, medical staff
may be afraid that relinquishing 'control' to patients might threaten their identity
(O' Flynn and Britten, 2006). A desire to retain this power imbalance has also been
demonstrated in nursing staff. Henderson (2003) interviewed nurses and found a
general consensus that they felt they 'know best', and that in general patients lacked
medical knowledge, requiring the nurses to retain their power and maintain control.
It is clear that such beliefs will be major barriers to patient involvement in safety initiatives. It is important therefore for health professionals to be aware of their beliefs
about participation, and the potential impact of such beliefs.

ACTIVITY 3.7   REFLECTION

Think about your own practice as a health professional, and consider the following
questions.

- How do you feel about patients getting involved in their safety?
- To date, how have you attempted to engage with patients about their safety?
- After reading this section, what approaches might you adopt in the future to
  encourage patient involvement?

This final section has focused on some ways in which you as a health professional
might encourage and support patients to become more involved both in the safety
of their own care, and that of others. It is clear that some of these approaches might
present you with more challenges than others, in terms of time, resources, even
threats to your identity as a health professional. Whatever these challenges, it is
useful to think about what approaches you might take to encourage patient involvement. Involving patients is now a policy and moral imperative – an imperative that
may just help you improve your practice and the safety of your patients.

Chapter summary

In this chapter we have demonstrated how and when patients might get involved
in the safety of themselves and others and discussed the relative benefits and
challenges of this involvement for patients, health professionals and healthcare

organisations. We presented evidence to suggest that patients might differ in terms of their willingness and ability to be involved in patient safety initiatives, and that this might change even for the same patient over time and the course of treatment. Lastly, we considered what practical steps you can take to encourage the involvement of patients in their safety.

Involving patients might be challenging to health professionals. To be a practitioner who encourages involvement you will need to be a good communicator and listener, who responds to feedback in a constructive way. You will need to take time to build relationships with patients – however brief their treatment – to invite and give credence to their involvement. However, the emerging evidence suggests that this approach is worthwhile, potentially reaping benefits for patients, health professionals and the healthcare organisations within which they work.

GOING FURTHER

A number of reviews about patient involvement in patient safety provide extra detail on some of the issues raised in this chapter:

- Longtin, Y, Sax, H, Leape, LL, Sheridan, SE, Donaldson, L and Pittet, D (2010) Patient participation: current knowledge and applicability to patient safety. *Mayo Clinic Proceedings,* 85: 53–62.

- Schwappach, DLB (2010) Engaging patients as vigilant partners in safety: a systematic review. *Medical Care Research and Review,* 67: 119–48.

There are also a number of organisations outside the health service that can be a useful source of information about patient involvement initiatives:

- The Clinical Human Factors Group is a broad coalition of healthcare professionals, managers and users of services who have partnered with experts in human factors from healthcare and other high-risk industries to campaign for change in the NHS: **www.chfg.org**.

- Action against Medical Accidents is an independent charity which promotes better patient safety and justice for people who have been affected by a medical accident: **www.avma.org.uk**.

chapter 4

Human Factors Engineering and Patient Safety

Peter Gardner

Achieving your medical degree

This chapter will help you to begin to meet the following requirements of *Tomorrow's Doctors* (General Medical Council, 2009a).

Outcome 2: The doctor as practitioner

The graduate will be able to:

19. Use information effectively in a medical context.

   (b) Make effective use of computers and other information systems, including storing and retrieving information.
   (d) Access information sources and use the information in relation to patient care, health promotion, giving advice and information to patients, and research and education.
   (e) Apply the principles, method and knowledge of health informatics to medical practice.

Outcome 3: The doctor as professional

The graduate will be able to:

23. Protect patients and improve care.

   (a) Place patients' needs and safety at the centre of the care process.
   (b) Deal effectively with uncertainty and change.
   (d) Promote, monitor and maintain health and safety in the clinical setting, understanding how errors can happen in practice, applying the principles of quality assurance, clinical governance and risk management to medical practice, and understanding responsibilities within the current systems for raising concerns about safety and quality.

Chapter overview

The world of modern healthcare is dominated by technology and it is important for doctors to understand the importance of their role in the correct and safe use of medical devices and information technology. Doctors (and other healthcare professionals) are the human components in a wider system that includes the devices and/or technology, and their role may be as consumers of information or operators of machinery. It follows that incorrect use or misunderstanding of technology may result in patient safety incidents and it is widely accepted that the likelihood of these incidents occurring is increased by poor design. Despite the existence of design methods to help ensure that devices and computer systems are both functional and usable, it is extremely difficult to design out all of the potential errors and usability issues that might occur, particularly taking into account the need to minimise the lead time for development. As a result, doctors who lack familiarity with certain devices will find that some are either difficult to use correctly or easy to use incorrectly. The interaction between human and system can therefore produce misunderstandings, incorrect actions or inappropriate use, with the potential for ineffective, unsafe or dangerous outcomes. Given that doctors do get involved in the design and procurement of equipment, an appreciation of the topics in this chapter may help both to improve designs and to ensure that poorly designed equipment is not purchased.

After reading this chapter you will be able to:

- understand the need for good design in the development and procurement of medical technology;
- discuss the potential types of error that can occur in the use of technology by doctors;
- outline methods that can be used to compare the usability of medical devices;
- develop an approach for your own learning about technology that you encounter in different clinical situations.

Introduction: what is human factors engineering and why is it relevant?

Human factors engineering is an activity that has its roots in the more general discipline of human factors, which is sometimes called ergonomics. In fact, this latter term may well be more familiar and you are probably already conjuring up images of 'ergonomically designed' consumer products that claim to be easier and more effective to use (e.g. can openers, pens, office chairs, mp3 players, mobile phones, computers – almost anything, in fact). One of the confusing things about the notion of 'ease of use' is that it can apply to both physical and logical characteristics of a product or device. For instance, we might be concerned about how easy something is to hold or manipulate, and so the shape and spatial location of features will be the focus. Alternatively we may be interested in whether the interaction between the product and the user is straightforward and understandable – something which is more relevant to electronic products or anything that provides information. You can see how this distinction between physical and logical characteristics applies to the consumer products listed above, but it also applies to the type of equipment that can be used in a medical setting, and we will return to this later.

Given this broad interpretation of the area, it might be useful to introduce a definition in order to understand a little more about what this chapter will cover. In the year 2000, the International Ergonomics Association approved the following definition for ergonomics, which serves as a good basis for understanding what human factors engineering is all about:

> *Ergonomics (or human factors) is the scientific discipline concerned with the understanding of the interactions among humans and other elements of a system, and the profession that applies theoretical principles, data and methods to design in order to optimize human well being and overall system performance.*
>
> *Practitioners of ergonomics, ergonomists, contribute to the planning, design and evaluation of tasks, jobs, products, organizations, environments and systems in order to make them compatible with the needs, abilities and limitations of people.*
>
> (International Ergonomics Association, 2000)

Concentrating on the second paragraph of this definition, it is clear that the use of technology takes place within a wider system that includes both organisational and individual factors. Figure 4.1 shows Carayon *et al.*'s (2006) conceptualisation of how these different factors might interact with each other in a clinical setting and affect the processes of care and patient outcomes.

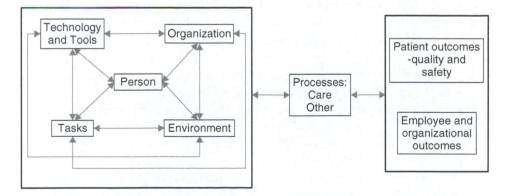

Figure 4.1 The system engineering initiative for patient safety (SEIPS) model of work system and patient safety. (Reproduced with permission from Carayon *et al.*, 2006.)

Central to the system engineering initiative for patient safety model is the fact that the person interacts with all the other elements but, in considering the role of technology, three things need to be considered:

1. the tasks that need to be performed;

2. the context within which they are being performed (environment and organisation);

3. the design of the technology being used.

The importance of tasks (e.g. procedures) and contexts (e.g. the environment on a ward) in terms of their effect on patient safety are beyond the scope of this chapter. The main aim is to raise your awareness of the design issues surrounding the correct and safe use of devices and computer systems and the potential implications for your own practice.

Case Studies: What's the evidence?

Consider these two examples described by Jacobson and Murray (2007):

1. A case in which two air tubes were mixed up. A patient on intensive care had a gastric tube (with slight suction) inserted in order to empty the stomach. The patient was also resting on a special mattress which is continually inflated and deflated in order to help prevent bedsores. A nurse noticed that the suction tube had become disconnected from the gastric tube but mistakenly attached the tube used for inflating the mattress. A nurse on the next shift noticed that the patient's abdomen was distended and was able to correct the problem with no harm done. It transpired that, although the two connections should not have been compatible, the mattress connection had earlier been broken and replaced by a simple piece of tubing that then allowed this error to occur.

2. A case in which an incubator for use with newborn babies began to overheat as a result of a short circuit. No alarm sounded because the design of the equipment meant that the short circuit effectively disconnected the alarm. The fact that the design of the incubator did not include a safety cut-out was of even more concern, and resulted in the incubator overheating to a temperature of 47°C. The purchasing procedure in the organisation did not include a routine inspection to ensure that the device complied with the relevant safety requirements. A nurse spotted the problem and prevented the baby coming to harm.

These examples neatly demonstrate the interaction between the technological and human components of the system. In the first, a well-meaning individual repaired part of the technology being used, but in so doing unwittingly created a violation of the safety feature that had been designed into the system. In the second, a poorly designed incubator malfunctioned and it was only the intervention of a nurse that stopped the incident having a serious or fatal outcome.

Why is the design of medical technology important?

You may be asking, why should I, as a medical student, be concerned about the design of the technology and devices used in healthcare? There are two reasons that you may find persuasive: firstly, that medical devices are an integral and ubiquitous feature of a doctor's working life, and secondly, that the number of patient safety incidents related to medical devices is increasing.

Medical devices are everywhere!

The wide diversity of equipment that is defined by the Medicines and Healthcare products Regulatory Agency (MHRA) as a 'medical device' includes everything from computerised tomography scanners to simple thermometers (Activity 4.1 and MHRA, 2011a). You should, therefore, appreciate the central role that medical devices and technology will play in your future career.

ACTIVITY 4.1

1. Access the document *Tomorrow's Doctors* (General Medical Council, 2009a) from the website of the General Medical Council, and go to *Appendix 1 – Practical procedures for graduates*. How many of the procedures listed here require the use of a medical device?
2. Access the document *Devices in Practice: A guide for professionals in health and social care* from the MHRA website (MHRA, 2011a). Go to section 4 and the related checklist at the end of the document that lists the common types of medical device. How familiar are you with the devices listed here? Are there any that you know are considered difficult to use by fellow students or nursing colleagues?

In considering the range of medical devices, it is important to make the distinction between more interactive devices and those which may be seen as medical tools. Both of these types of device are a form of medical technology and their design should take account of the human factors that could affect their successful implementation and use.

Interactive devices have an interface (controls, buttons for entering information, screens or displays of information) and examples are drug infusion pumps, blood pressure monitors and electrocardiograph machines. Medical tools include a myriad of devices such as syringes, needles, cannulae, blood containers and catheters.

Surprisingly, there is a degree of overlap between the human factors issues that are relevant for these different types of device. For instance, it is often helpful if the design of a device exploits the expectations of how it might work. In other words, there should be some consistency between the operation of different types of blood pressure monitor, or in the connection between different syringes and needles. If there is inconsistency between different models of device, then it is possible that a particular piece of equipment could be set up and used incorrectly because the clinician has based his or her understanding of how to use it on an experience with another machine. At the very least, if you are not familiar with the operation of a piece of equipment, then the time taken to perform a particular procedure will be lengthened and you may not look very professional from the patient's perspective.

Equally, the ease of handling or manipulation of a device should be considered from the human perspective. For instance, the buttons on an interactive device should be easy to operate. If the controls of a device are too small or too close together, then there is the possibility that incorrect information will be entered or that the device will be set up incorrectly. With regard to more practical procedures, it should, for example, be easy to manipulate the components of different systems that can be used to take blood samples.

ACTIVITY 4.2

Use an internet search engine to search for short videos showing the use of the Vacutainer and Monovette systems for sampling blood (there are several available on YouTube). Make short notes about the sequence of actions that need to take place. What are the key differences and similarities? Do any elements of these procedures have the potential to compromise patient safety?

This activity demonstrates that, although a great deal of care can be taken in the design and production of different device designs, the lack of consistency and differences in the way that components should be handled may produce problems for practitioners who are unfamiliar with all the alternatives. It is therefore important to prepare yourself adequately to cope with these variations.

Errors arising from the use of medical devices are increasing

The frequency of reports of adverse incidents that relate to medical devices is increasing. In a recent report about adverse incidents due to medical devices, the MHRA states that it received information about more than 10,000 incidents during 2010, which represented an increase of 13 per cent compared to the previous year and an increase of 42 per cent compared to ten years previously (MHRA, 2011b).

What's the evidence?

The National Patient Safety Agency (NPSA) publishes quarterly data summaries that show more detailed analysis of the types of incident that are reported to the National Reporting and Learning Service. The most recent data available on device incidents show that, between April 2006 and March 2007, there were 326 individual device incidents that led to severe harm or death of the patient (NPSA, 2008). Figure 4.2 shows the breakdown of the incident types and that just over a quarter of these may have had an element of user error or poor design.

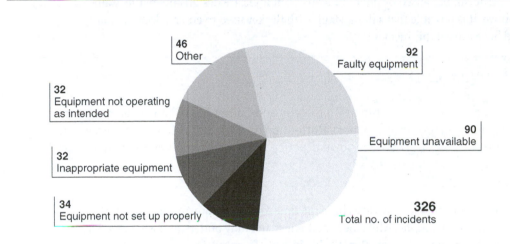

Figure 4.2 Most frequently reported incident types (device-related incidents) in England and Wales from April 2006 to March 2007. (Source: National Patient Safety Agency, 2008.)

Ward and Clarkson (2007) point out that, when presenting statistics, such as these presented by the MHRA, it is not always possible to represent the underlying reasons for the incidents fully. For instance, it is not absolutely clear whether incidents classified as 'equipment not operating as intended' or 'equipment not set up properly' are due to poor design features that have allowed or facilitated incorrect use, or because of errors on the part of the person responsible for operating the device. Such user errors may have occurred as a result of insufficient training, a lack of familiarity with the equipment or a misunderstanding about whether the device was functioning correctly.

It follows that there will be some incidents in which it is hard to determine whether poor design has led to an error by the user. In other words, if a piece of equipment is poorly designed and someone uses it incorrectly, we may not be able to determine which is to blame – the equipment or the person operating it.

The NPSA (2008) report cites an example of an incident that occurred with a syringe driver which was categorised as 'equipment not operating as intended':

> *On checking progress of syringe driver at 22:00, I discovered the syringe empty. The syringe driver was commenced at 15:00 hours to run over 24 hours and should be set to run at 2mls per hour but was set at 20mls per hour. The syringe driver contained diamorphine 30mg and cyclizine 100mg. The patient was receiving this for pain control in palliative care.*
>
> (NPSA, 2008, p16)

It is not obvious from this example how the syringe driver came to be set up incorrectly but one possibility is that the numbers were keyed in incorrectly. Although one might expect the entry of such crucial information to be given high attention and checked, as Thimbleby and Cairns (2010) demonstrated, the possibility of a number entry error can be caused by poor or inconsistent interface design and, in the example above, it is possible that a design fault with the key used to enter a decimal point could have caused this incident.

ACTIVITY 4.3

Access the paper written by Thimbleby and Cairns (2010) and read sections 1 and 2 (this is a free-access paper). Reflect on how the potential for errors in entering numbers might affect your own practice. How might you ensure that you are less likely to make such errors?

It seems obvious that if individuals have the time to concentrate on what they are doing, are not interrupted while they are doing it and fully understand what it is that they are supposed to be doing, then the likelihood of committing such number entry errors will be reduced. Equally, it is important to realise that medical technology is increasingly subject to good design methods. There is a great deal of activity that is going on to ensure that both interactive devices and medical tools are fit for purpose and safe to use. In the next section we consider the notion of the design cycle and the importance of the user in ensuring that these aims are met.

Design and usability of technology

As a medical student, you may have already had experience of the wide variety of devices, equipment and software with which you will need to interact on a daily basis. Some of the technology that you encounter will strike you as being completely amazing in terms of its sophistication and scientific roots. Other technology may be less impressive, but in all cases you will want it to be as easy and as safe to use as possible. In this section, we will look at two basic principles that underlie the development of new technology and that contribute to the overall goal of ensuring that technology meets its needs: the notions of user-centred design and usability.

User-centred design and usability

Typically, the design cycle (for almost any product) comprises a series of stages. Rogers *et al.* (2011) identify four stages as typical in the design of interactive products but these stages are equally applicable to the variety of medical devices that we are considering.

1. Establishing requirements – this stage requires consultation with all the stakeholders involved in a project to identify what needs have to be met by the new design. It is important to establish what kind of people will be using the end product and in what context. What functions must be performed, how quickly and to what level or standard, and to what extent must usability constraints be met? It may be necessary to use multiple and diverse methods to derive requirements, because users often find it difficult to verbalise their requirements. This may be because they do not have sufficient experience of the capabilities and constraints of the intended technology.

2. Designing alternatives – this is the creative or innovative stage in which different solutions are developed in order to meet the requirements. There are a number of different ways in which design solutions can be produced. These might involve end users as part of the process or may require a design team to work together separately.

3. Prototyping – the fidelity, or likeness to reality, of prototypes may increase as the design matures. Early in the prototyping phase, ideas may simply be realised on paper as a form of 'storyboard' which sketches the nature of an interaction or as a three-dimensional computer-aided design drawing. Later in the design cycle prototypes may become more physically similar to the final implementation.

4. Evaluating – it is important that prototypes are evaluated against the original requirements throughout the design cycle using an iterative loop of design–implement–test. Two or three iterations should result in a final implementation for evaluation and release. In e-health interventions, Catwell and Sheikh (2009) advocate a continuous cycle of systematic evaluation to take place at all stages of development. They argue that policy decisions should be based on the evidence gained from such evaluation rather than other factors, such as *industry lobbying, political expediency, or enthusiasm to implement technology simply because it exists* (Catwell and Sheikh, 2009, p5).

User-centred design

Arguably, the most important element running through the stages described above is the role of the user in shaping the design. The unavoidable conclusion is that technology should be required to fit to the needs of the user, rather than the user being required to fit to the needs of the technology. This principle drove the development of the user-centred design movement during the 1980s (Norman and Draper, 1986) and was initially applied to the design of computer interfaces with the simple aim of making them easier to use (or more user-friendly).

More recently, the notion of user-centredness has pervaded many domains of design, including web pages, electronic devices, consumer products, buildings and, of course, medical technology. The central tenet of the approach is that the user should be involved in the design process from the very start. The expectation is that the development of a new product should follow a structured design lifecycle like the one shown above, but that the user should be involved in most, if not all, of that process. At the end of the process the final product should be evaluated against the requirements that were originally derived from the intended user and one way in which a design may be evaluated is to assess whether it is easy to use. Bate and Robert (2006) suggest that the principle of involving users has been less frequently applied when designing for healthcare compared to designing for other domains. They argue that there is scope for patients, in particular, to have greater participation in co-designing systems and services for healthcare.

Usability

We often refer to the 'usability' of a product, device or interface as being a quality that can be compared between alternatives, the implication being that we will prefer options that are more 'usable' than others. It is perhaps important to highlight the distinction made at the beginning of the chapter between the physical characteristics and logical characteristics of a product or device, and remember that both of these dimensions may contribute to the overall perception of usability. Devices that are fiddly, unwieldy or complex in terms of their physical attributes will be considered less usable, as will those that have interfaces that are difficult to understand, or that have multiple modes and complex sequences of operation.

The concept of usability therefore seems to be an important issue in considering the design of medical devices and the implications for patient safety, but is it possible to be more precise about how it might be measured or assessed?

The International Organization for Standardization defines usability as the: *extent to which a product can be used by specified users to achieve specified goals with effectiveness, efficiency and satisfaction in a specified context of use* (International Organization for Standardization, 1998).

Here the usability of the device clearly depends on the performance and opinion of users following their experience of using the device. In a medical setting we might ask how we could approach measuring each of the elements in this definition in order to allow comparison between competitor devices. A particular model of device will be deemed 'usable' if the people who are meant to use it are able to perform all the necessary tasks accurately (effectiveness), in an appropriate amount of time (efficiency) without frustration, confusion or uncertainty (satisfaction).

What's the evidence?

A research paper by Fairbanks et al. (2007) compared the usability of two defibrillators commonly used in practice with the aim of identifying any hazards that might arise from their use. You can view these two machines online. They are the Life Pak10 (www.physio-control.com/support/technical-support-faq/index.aspx?id= 2436) and the LifePak12 (www.physio-control.com/ProductDetail.aspx?id=546).

Participants comprised 14 paramedics who used the two devices in four different simulated scenarios. Both quantitative and qualitative data were gathered and it was found that, although one device was reported to be easier to learn, the other was considered to be more effective in an emergency and generally easier to use.

The effectiveness and efficiency with which a device may be used can clearly be measured objectively (e.g. number of errors committed, or time taken to perform a task) but such measures are most appropriate in a controlled or simulated environment and may prove difficult to gather in a field setting such as healthcare. More commonly, usability is measured using subjective questionnaire-based measures. There are a number of different measures that are available to use but some are rather long and, again, may be difficult to use in a field setting. One measure that is quick and easy to use is the System Usability Scale (SUS) developed by Brooke (1996). The SUS has been empirically evaluated (Bangor et al., 2008) and has been used in a healthcare setting (Sawka et al., 2011). Although this measure was designed to be used to evaluate computer interfaces, it could easily be adapted for use with other types of equipment that fall into the category of medical devices. The strength of using a standardised measure like the SUS is that it allows direct comparison between competing alternatives and the score obtained for an individual system also gives some indication as to whether an acceptable level of usability has been achieved (Bangor et al., 2008).

ACTIVITY 4.4

Bangor et al. (2008) present an updated version of the original SUS, first developed by Brooke (1996). The ten statements from Bangor and colleagues are shown below and have been further adapted for use in this activity.

Use the SUS to assess a medical device. This could be one that is regularly used on a ward or perhaps an over-the-counter device that you have purchased for your own use, e.g. blood pressure monitor, blood glucose monitor. Alternatively, if you do not have access to a suitable device, you could use a website that is unfamiliar to you, e.g. for booking a train journey, or purchasing your weekly shopping.

Each statement must be rated on a 5-point scale from 1= strongly disagree to 5 = strongly agree.

1. I think that I would like to use this device/website frequently.
2. I found the device/website unnecessarily complex.
3. I thought the device/website was easy to use.
4. I think that I would need the support of a technical person to be able to use this device/website.

5. I found that the various functions in this device/website were well integrated.
6. I thought that there was too much inconsistency in this device/website.
7. I would imagine that most people would learn to use this device/website very quickly.
8. I found the device/website very awkward to use.
9. I felt very confident using the device/website.
10. I needed to learn a lot of things before I could get going with this device/website.

The SUS score is derived by summing all the responses to the ten questions and then multiplying by 2.5. Bangor *et al.* (2008) suggest that a score above 70 indicates that the usability is acceptable, whereas below 50 indicates that it is not acceptable. Scores in the range 50–70 are marginal.

This section has indicated how the process of designing new technology may best be approached, by taking a user-centred design perspective, and has considered how we may gather data from users to allow us to assess the usability of devices that are being developed or are already in existence. However, there are also known design principles that should be used to inform the design of equipment and the next section outlines the key ideas and shows that it is possible to assess design quality by reviewing particular devices against such principles.

Design principles and heuristic review

Earlier a distinction was made between medical devices that can be seen as tools and those which have interactive features. It was pointed out that, at a general level, there is some overlap between the design principles that are important to consider for both types of device. For instance, consistency of use is a principle that might apply to both types of device, although there are also more specific principles which we will consider here.

First, with regard to medical tools, it is important that devices are intuitive in their use. An intuitive design is often referred to as a design that has 'affordance', or in other words a design that 'affords' a particular use. A good non-medical example might be a saw used for cutting wood. Even if you have never used a saw before, it is obvious how it should be held and which is the 'business end'. In other words, in the medical domain it should be possible for a healthcare professional (or student!) with little experience of a particular device to work out what the device is used for and what the key components are, although it is always important to make sure that the correct training has been given before using an unfamiliar device. Nevertheless, it is likely that you will find that there are packs of medical equipment (e.g. cannulae, infusion sets) that are not that intuitive to use, and that will provide a challenge as to how they should be connected together and used correctly.

A second design principle with regard to medical tools concerns the need to take account of human physical limitations. The field of anthropometry concerns the normal dimensions of human beings and the range of movement that they can engage in. A good example would be to ensure that components are not too small to be manipulated, or too stiff to be moved into the correct position.

Other design principles might include the need for components to be easily visible, labelled clearly, and if appropriate, using a consistent system of colour coding.

The following case study demonstrates how a serious patient safety incident prompted the design and production of new equipment in order to help stop similar errors occurring.

Case Study: Wrong route delivery of vincristine

In 2001 a teenager called Wayne Jowett was receiving treatment for cancer. A chemotherapy medicine, vincristine, was injected via the wrong route and resulted in his death. It should be noted that vincristine is a medicine that should only be injected intravenously, but on this occasion it was administered intrathecally (via the spinal route). If injected into the spine it is normally fatal.

A detailed investigation by Professor Brian Toft took place. If you are interested, you can read the report, which is published on the Department of Health website (Toft, 2001). One of the key outcomes of the report was that it had been possible to fit a standard Luer-compatible syringe to the spinal needle that had been inserted into Wayne Jowett's spine. The Luer-compatible syringe is also used for intravenous administration and in this case contained a drug that should not be administered intrathecally. As a result one of the recommendations of the report was that:

> A new spinal needle with a connection that cannot fit Luer mount intravenous syringes should be introduced, in conjunction with a new syringe which can only be fitted to that specific spinal needle.

> (Toft, 2001, p48)

Following publication of the report, work has been ongoing to investigate the feasibility of designing and implementing a new spinal connector system that can only be used for intrathecal procedures. This new design should provide an engineered solution to act as a physical barrier to prevent this type of error occurring.

Approximately ten years on from the death of Wayne Jowett, the NPSA issued a Patient Safety Alert (NPSA/2011/PSA001) stating that:

By 1 April 2012 healthcare organisations should have completed actions to ensure that all spinal (intrathecal) bolus doses and lumbar puncture samples are performed using syringes, needles and other devices with connectors that cannot also connect with intravenous equipment.

(NPSA, 2011)

A number of manufacturers indicated an intention to produce re-designed connectors in order to meet this need.

Some of the key issues involved in designing and implementing these solutions are provided in Lawton *et al.* (2009) and it is important that you read this paper to understand the need for good design in this type of equipment.

The discussion now turns to the design principles that are important in more interactive medical devices. Following on from our previous consideration of the methods used to develop computer systems and interfaces, it is important to understand the key design principles, or heuristics, that define usability in interactive devices. Jakob Nielsen (1994) developed a list of such principles that are widely accepted as providing a guideline for system developers. However, it is probably worth noting that the number of principles in the list has varied over the years (from 10 to 14), and also that there are many instances in the literature where researchers have tailored Nielsen's basic list for use in different domains (e.g. websites, mobile applications, even building design). It is perhaps beyond the scope of this book (and your interest) to go through all of the principles, but we might consider a couple of useful examples.

1. Visibility of system status – it should be possible for the user to understand what state the system is currently in, based on feedback provided by the system. For instance, using a domestic example, it can be important to understand when a video recorder is in standby mode. Many older devices required the recorder to be in standby mode for a preset recording to work. If the device was left on, the recording would not take place, even though the timer had been set. It is highly likely that this error would have occurred because the difference between the two modes was not sufficiently visible to the user (at least, that is the excuse I used with my wife!).

2. Consistency and standards – terms and actions in the system should be consistently used. For example, a symbol should not mean two different things depending on where it appears in the interaction. It is quite common for the symbol 'X' to be used in different ways in software. For instance, 'X' might mean that a particular window will be closed, or it might mean that something will be deleted or

it might mean that something is selected. Consistency is also important between different (competitor) products that may be used in a hospital. If a 'big red button' turns one machine on, but a similar button turns a machine from a different manufacturer off, then there could clearly be confusion for an inexperienced user.

Nielsen suggests that any device can be assessed in terms of how well it meets the principles in a process known as heuristic review. The idea is that a small group of experienced individuals interact with the device and generate a list of usability problems (categorised by each of the principles). They then assign a severity rating to each problem which takes into account the frequency, impact and persistence of the problem. An excellent example of how this technique has been used in a medical setting is provided in a paper by Zhang *et al.* (2003). This paper demonstrates that it is possible to use this technique to compare different devices and make a judgment about which device is likely to produce more errors in its use.

What's the evidence?

Zhang *et al.* (2003) use the technique of heuristic review to perform a comparison between two infusion pumps. They demonstrate that the technique helps to uncover key differences between the devices in terms of the number and severity of the usability problems encountered. They conclude that it is possible to use heuristic review to make judgments about the relative likelihood of patient safety problems occurring as a result of using different systems. This kind of knowledge would allow relevant training to be put in place to ameliorate such problems, or might affect purchasing choices. It should also provide manufacturers with specific recommendations to enable improvement in the design of their products.

In addition, Chan *et al.* (2011) conducted a heuristic review of what they term a computerised provider order entry system (CPOE: also known as computerised physician/prescriber order entry system). They focused on a component of the system which allows the creation of standardised sets of medication orders in order to improve the efficiency and accuracy of medication ordering. Their paper again highlights the usefulness of the heuristic review technique and in particular recommends that a heuristic review should be conducted early in the product-prototyping phase. Another feature of the Chan *et al.* paper is that they included a trained clinician as part of their review team and found that 62 per cent of the usability violations were exclusively identified by this individual. This highlights the importance of having an individual with relevant knowledge of the topic area as part of the review team.

The process of heuristic review takes a slightly different perspective on the assessment of usability than the one discussed earlier in this section. Measurement of usability can either be focused on the user, in the sense that data are collected from people who are likely to use the system, or it can make use of experts with knowledge of good design principles to provide a judgment on the design of a system. However, what seems clear from the evidence presented above is that there is much to be gained from including people with knowledge of a particular context in the technique of heuristic review.

ACTIVITY 4.5

Go to the following webpage, which is part of Jakob Nielsen's UseIt website: **www. useit.com/alertbox/20050411.html**. The title of the piece is 'Medical Usability: How to Kill Patients Through Bad Design'. Read Nielsen's commentary on the paper by Koppel *et al.* (2005) in which an analysis of a CPOE system revealed 22 ways in which the system could lead to increased risk of medication error. You may also like to access the original paper in order to get extra detail. Nielsen's main point is that most of the reported flaws in the CPOE system concern usability problems that have been well known in the human factors literature for many years. Reflect on whether the technique of heuristic review would have uncovered these problems so that they could be addressed as part of the normal design cycle. How important would it be to have reviewers with relevant clinical knowledge in order to uncover these errors?

Finally, it must be pointed out that the NPSA has produced a set of detailed guidelines for testing medical devices (NPSA, 2010) and the topics of user-centred design, usability and heuristic review are among those that are discussed in more detail than has been possible here.

Chapter summary

In this final short section, it is important to stand back from the principles, techniques and evidence that have been presented in this chapter and return to the issues that we suggested make an appreciation of human factors issues important for a medical student and soon-to-be junior doctor. These issues were firstly, that medical devices are an important and ubiquitous element of the clinical setting and secondly, that errors relating to medical device usage are on the increase.

This chapter acknowledged that the use of the human factors engineering approach assumes that technology is part of a wider system that includes human and other organisational factors. However, we focused on the way in which technology is designed and the impact that this might have for interaction with humans.

We examined the need for good design methods and principles and considered methods for assessing the relationship between the design of the device and the potential for patient safety incidents. It is clear that, despite efforts to encourage

---

and promote good design, there is still a risk of harmful patient safety incidents where examples of poor design exist. As a medical student, you may not feel that you are in a position to do much about poorly designed devices and equipment but there are a number of principles that would be helpful to bear in mind when working in a clinical setting.

- Be aware of your own limitations and of the limitations of the technology – you are only human, and therefore you are subject to the problems that poor design can bring.
- Do not assume that you know how to do everything – try to gain experience of different devices and equipment in low-risk situations. Ask for training and consult more experienced colleagues if you are not sure.
- Conform to the correct procedures for using devices.
- Report any faulty equipment and don't be scared to question if you think that something is not quite right.
- Raise any concerns about the usability of a device with a senior colleague.

GOING FURTHER

Jacobson, J and Murray, A (2007) *Medical Devices: Use and safety*. Edinburgh: Churchill Livingstone.
This is a very interesting book that deals with the kinds of error that can occur with medical devices. It is organised in a structured way and is really a collection of case studies, some of which are very disturbing.

Norris, B (2011) Systems human factors: how far have we come? *BMJ Quality and Safety*, published online 7 November 2011.
From the journal *BMJ Quality and Safety*, this is a recent and short opinion piece from the NPSA about the importance of systems human factors for our understanding of the design and implementation of technology in the clinical setting. This is a useful read and sets the current position in context.

Shortliffe, E (2010) Biomedical informatics in the education of physicians. *Journal of the American Medical Association*, 304(11): 1227–8.
A short, thought-provoking commentary which is directly relevant for medical students and highlights the need for educating physicians in the use of information, as well as education in basic and clinical science.

Wiklund, M, Kendler, J and Strochlic, AY (2011) *Usability testing of medical devices*. Boca Raton, FL: CRC Press.
This book provides a practical introduction on how to conduct usability testing with medical devices.

chapter 5

How to be a Creative and Innovative Practitioner

Angela Grange, Valerie Rhodes and Ann Starkey

Achieving your medical degree

This chapter will help you to meet the following requirements of *Tomorrow's Doctors* (General Medical Council, 2009a).

Outcome 3: The doctor as a professional

The graduate will be able to:

21. Reflect, learn and teach others:

   [A] Acquire, assess, apply and integrate new knowledge, learn to adapt to changing circumstances and ensure that patients receive the highest level of professional care.

   (c) Continually and systematically reflect on practice and, whenever necessary, translate that reflection into action, using improvement techniques and audit appropriately – for example, by critically appraising the prescribing of others.

22. Learn and work effectively within a multiprofessional team:

   [A] Understand and respect the roles and expertise of health and social care professionals in the context of working and learning as a multiprofessional team.
   [B] Understand the contribution that effective interdisciplinary team working makes to the delivery of safe and high-quality care.

23. Protect patients and improve care:

   [A] Place patients' needs and safety at the centre of the care process.
   [B] Deal effectively with uncertainty and change.

Chapter overview

Front-line staff, such as junior doctors and nurses, want to provide the best possible care for patients, using the latest treatment and the latest technologies. Innovations in healthcare are essential for the development of these treatments and technologies. Given the current financial climate, and population growth pressures that healthcare organisations are facing, doing things differently to achieve the same quality of care, or better quality of care for less, is becoming the norm. Innovation has a vital role to play if we are to continue to improve patient outcomes, deliver value-for-money services and also boost the national economy.

The NHS is full of brilliant people with brilliant ideas to change healthcare for the better, but these individuals need support to take their ideas forward, test them, refine them and then get them into everyday practice to benefit patients as quickly as possible (NHS Chief Executive, 2011). This chapter provides an introduction to innovation in healthcare and aims to stimulate your thinking about your role in this process, including how to be creative and innovative. We focus on the less tangible kind of innovations, those which improve services offered to patients either through different ways of service delivery or new innovative services. For information on more tangible types of innovations such as devices, designs, copyright, trademarks and software, and how to exploit these types of innovations, please refer to the government's Intellectual Property Officer's website: **www.ipo.gov.uk.** The chapter is intentionally written in a user-friendly way focusing on tools and techniques you may want to use within and outside your placements. There are additional references and resources you may want to access that provide the evidence for some of the approaches that we advocate here, with further reading suggested at the end.

After reading this chapter you will be able to:

- identify the attributes of an innovative individual;
- describe what innovation in healthcare means and why it is relevant to you and the NHS;
- discuss tools and techniques to help generate innovative ideas;
- identify the considerations for a successful innovation.

Introduction: what is innovation in healthcare?

There are many definitions of innovation and there is often blurring between the terms 'innovation', 'invention' and 'improvement'. For the purposes of this chapter we will use the definitions overleaf, but any search will produce many more.

Innovation, Invention, Improvement

Innovation is an idea, service or product new to the NHS, or applied in a way that is new to healthcare, which significantly improves the quality of health and care wherever it is applied (NHS Chief Executive, 2011).

Invention is concerned with the generation of new ideas which have the potential to make someone or something better and which did not exist previously (Plamping et al., 2009).

Improvement is any method that brings about a measurable benefit against a stated aim (Granville, 2006).

In this context, invention is the creation of a new product or service stemming from an individual's idea. Before it can be shared and taken up in practice or for wider-scale general use, the idea will need to be nurtured and developed, involving different people with different expertise. Innovation, on the other hand, is the successful introduction of a service or product that is new to the organisation in question. It may have been imported from another healthcare organisation or it may have come from a different industry and be entirely new to the NHS. Innovation thus consists of three stages: (1) invention (as defined above); (2) adoption (including prototyping and evaluation), which is the testing of new ways of doing things and putting this into practice; and (3) diffusion (or spread), which is the systematic uptake or copying of an innovation across the service (NHS Chief Executive, 2011). A discussion of adoption and diffusion is beyond the remit of this chapter, but will be discussed briefly in the next chapter. We do, however, refer you to further reading about these aspects of innovation at the end of the chapter.

Why do we need to innovate?

We live in a technology-driven world where the pace of change is rapid and where failing to keep up with modern technology means being left behind. The success of human beings as a species owes much to our ability to adapt and find new ways of meeting the challenges of our changing environment, in short, to be innovative.

Innovation can be driven by the need to meet socioeconomic challenges, such as the development of technology and materials to enable the construction of high-rise buildings as a solution to accommodate the increasing numbers of people living in cities. It can also come from a need to adapt to economic or customer demands. Examples include the use of computer technology adapted from the business world to medicine, where it can be used to help monitor people's safety in their own homes, or using Twitter as a social network to keep patients up to date with healthcare initiatives. NHS Direct is now available as an application (app) for mobile phones to improve accessibility and reach more users. Through postcodes or a global positioning system (GPS), the app can identify the user's location and provide directions to the nearest accident and emergency department. The NHS is exploiting this technology for a number of reasons, including accessibility of services, targeting services at a particular age group and responding to new and emerging ways of communication, ever mindful of improving cost-effectiveness. We should – and therefore do – innovate to meet the challenges of our changing environment. In the field of healthcare, this is becoming increasingly important as healthcare systems around the world struggle to cope with an ever-growing elderly population at a time of global economic recession.

Who can be innovative?

Organisations don't innovate – people do!
(Dr Stephen Lundin, author of the FISH! philosophy, 2008)

It is clear when looking at innovations in the healthcare system that many have come from those staff on the ground, people working every day to resolve complex issues, making important decisions, listening to the concerns of their patients and often seeing innovative solutions to the challenges they face. The importance of staff coming up with ideas was highlighted when the Google founders Brin and Page discovered that innovative ideas progressed more quickly if they came directly from and were executed by their staff, rather than being backed by them (Amabile and Khaire, 2008). This also raises another point about the importance of leadership in the development of an innovation by engaging with the right people at the right time to the right degree to allow creativity to flourish (Amabile and Khaire, 2008).

Innovation can be *incremental* in that it builds on existing practice; it can create a completely new way of doing something, a *radical change*; or it can completely revolutionise the way things are done and therefore be *disruptive*. It can occur on a large scale or small scale. Innovation can occur through a number of routes, via the delivery or management of patient care, in education or training, or through a research and development project or programme. Innovation may fall into some of the following categories:

- a new treatment;
- a new device;
- new drugs;
- software;
- training materials;
- treatment protocols;
- new systems and processes, such as a new assessment tool, training package or handover process.

ACTIVITY 5.1

Drawing upon your own experience in clinical practice, think of an example of an innovation for each category in the table below. You may want to think about examples of small-scale innovations developed locally in a ward, department or healthcare organisation where you have worked recently or large-scale innovations developed and implemented on a wider scale throughout the NHS. You may even have an idea of your own.

Innovation category	Example
A new treatment	
A new device	
A new drug	
New software	
Training materials	
Treatment protocol	
New system or process	

Qualities of an innovator

Everyone can come up with new and exciting ideas, but not everyone can take that idea and make it a reality. So what makes those individuals different? Many of us will have worked with people we would describe as being genuinely innovative, people who have led new ideas in their field and who have changed how care is provided.

There are certain qualities or traits we can all adopt which will enable us to be more open to new concepts, ideas and creative approaches – and therefore more likely to come up with innovative ideas. Some of these qualities are listed below.

- Be curious: constantly ask questions to help you understand the issues and challenges more fully.

- Bring in new ideas and 'horizon scan' for new technologies and systems from inside and outside the health system.

- Innovators do not innovate in total isolation; you need to be able to work collaboratively with others and 'let go' of your idea so others can contribute and take it further.

- Be a good listener – really listen to those around you – the views and concerns of patients, service users and junior staff at the front end who may have the solutions.

- Do not be afraid to challenge the status quo and try different approaches, take 'positive risks' and do not be afraid to learn from your mistakes.

- Have a passion for what you are doing.

- Have the humility to know that you do not always have the answers.

- Remain positive-minded and see problems as challenges with solutions waiting to be found.

The traits of successful innovators are described in numerous books and articles and correspond with the qualities above. The innovation theorist Clay Christensen, in *The Innovator's DNA* (Christensen *et al.*, 2011), outlines the five qualities that he believes every innovator needs to possess:

1. associating and connecting – being able to draw connections between problems and ideas that may be based in unrelated fields;

2. questioning – asking questions that challenge the usual way of doing things and the reasoning behind decisions;

3. observing – scrutinising the behaviour and actions of others and identifying ways of doing things differently;

4. networking – meeting with people from different backgrounds with different views and perspectives;

5. experimenting – trying out interactive experiments and provoking responses to achieve new insights and ideas.

Case Study

We provide as a case study an example of a patient safety innovation where the innovator demonstrated the associating and connecting quality described above.

Atul Gawande, a US surgeon, was concerned at the number of errors taking place across operating theatres in his hospital. When he looked in detail at what caused the errors he found failures that were avoidable but yet common and persistent.

He *associated* the numbers of errors with the complex nature of medicine, its innumerable interventions, the numbers of practitioners involved, the amount of things that can go wrong. In summary, he concluded: *the volume and complexity of what we know has exceeded our individual ability to deliver its benefits correctly, safely, or reliably. Knowledge has both saved us and burdened us.*

He *connected* with other industries that also faced the challenges of complexity and the need to maintain a low failure rate – the aviation and construction industries. He found that they reduced and managed failure by the use of checklists and, as he spent time with a chief engineer to look at this process in more detail, he made a further connection, that the systems within a building were in fact similar to that of a human body. He then realised that the use of checklists to reduce failures could also apply in healthcare (Gawande, 2011).

Initially the checklist approach to safety was applied and tested locally and then in June 2008 the World Health Organization (WHO) launched the Safe Surgery Saves Lives programme which included the surgical safety checklist. Between October 2007 and September 2009, the WHO Safe Surgery Saves Lives study group carried out research across eight hospitals in eight cities around the world (including St Mary's Hospital, London), representing high-, middle- and low-income countries. The group studied 3,733 patients before implementation of the checklist and 3,955 patients after implementation of the checklist, studying the rate of complications during hospitalisation, including death, within the first 30 days after the operation.

The study showed that, with the use of a checklist, surgical complications were reduced by more than one-third and deaths by almost one-half (Haynes *et al.*, 2009). On the basis of the findings from this study, the National Patient Safety Agency (NPSA), in collaboration with a professional expert reference group, adapted the checklist for use in England and Wales. In 2009, the NPSA issued a patient safety alert requiring all healthcare organisations to implement the WHO surgical safety checklist for every patient undergoing a surgical procedure (NPSA/2009/PSA002/U1).

ACTIVITY 5.2

Think about your recent clinical placement and an area of practice that caused you concern or you felt was a patient safety issue, e.g. medicines management, delivery of an aspect of patient care, communication with colleagues. Write down this concern or issue in a few sentences in the box below. Then choose one of the qualities of innovators from the list above (associating and connecting, questioning, observing, networking and experimenting) and write down your thoughts on how you will apply this quality to investigate your patient safety issue. For example, if your patient safety issue is around the management of medicines for patients on discharge from hospital, you may want to choose the questioning attribute and question nurses, pharmacists and doctors as to why they follow the procedures that they do when managing discharge medications.

My patient safety issue:

My chosen innovation attribute:

How I plan to apply this attribute to investigate my patient safety issue:

Creative thinking

Imagination is more important than knowledge. For knowledge is limited, whereas imagination embraces the entire world, stimulating progress, giving birth to evolution.

(Albert Einstein, 1931)

Innovative ideas can come to mind in an inspirational moment, but sometimes we need a more planned and purposeful approach, especially if we want to generate a large number of ideas to address a specific issue or problem. Paul Plsek, the author of *Creativity, Innovation and Quality*, calls this approach 'directed creativity' (Plsek, 1997). He describes a directed creativity cycle in four phases (Figure 5.1):

1. preparation, in which careful observation and analysis take place;

2. imagination, in which ideas are generated and harvested;

3. development, in which those ideas are enhanced and evaluated;

4. action, which is the end result of the idea being implemented.

We will use the four phases as a framework for the rest of this chapter and we have included tools and exercises that you can try out for yourself. To help you get the most from this process we suggest you identify an issue, challenge or problem that you may have experienced in a recent clinical placement or experience and to which you wish to apply a solution. Then use this example in the exercises that follow. You may wish to capture your identified issue in the space below as a reminder of what you are aiming to improve.

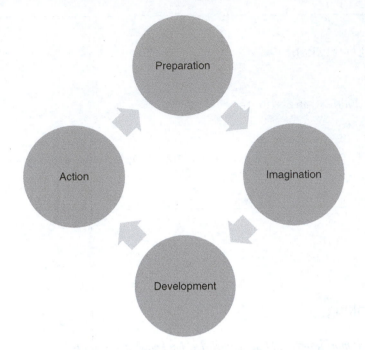

Figure 5.1 Directed creativity cycle (based on the ideas of Plsek, 1997).

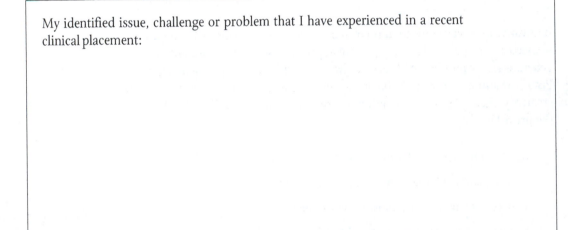

My identified issue, challenge or problem that I have experienced in a recent clinical placement:

Preparation

The quality of creative ideas depends on the quality of the preparation that went into them.

(Plsek, 1997)

Preparation is the point before we even start to engage in the process of creating ideas or solutions, the point at which we clarify what we are trying to do and ask the important questions: who, what, when, where and why? Good preparation enables a better understanding of the issue or challenge considered. The NHS Institute for Innovation and Improvements' *Thinking Differently* guide (Maher *et al.*, 2010) calls this phase 'Stop Before You Start', describing it as a period of reflection, a framing of the issue and looking at ways of reframing it to enable different ways of thinking. Paul Plsek identifies preparation as an essential requirement in generating ideas and sees what is generated from this phase as the raw materials that are required for the development of innovative concepts (Plsek, 1997).

Much of this phase is mental preparation and could involve observing what is happening, or collecting data from research or audits, reading information from wide-ranging fields or possibly talking to others from non-related areas. All the findings should be noted so you have records of the process. Both Plsek (**www.directed creativity.com**) and the *Thinking Differently* toolkit (Maher *et al.*, 2010) provide tools that can help you in this phase. A useful tool that you may want to use is Edward de Bono's six thinking hats, based on the principle of parallel thinking – everyone thinking in the same direction, from the same perspective, at the same time. It helps people step outside the confines of fixed positions and one way of thinking. Western thinking style is based on adversarial debate: people thinking and interacting from differing perspectives and positions. This tool enables us to look at things in a collaborative way, beyond our normal perspective, to see new opportunities. For more information about how to use this tool, go to **www.institute.nhs.uk**.We have selected a tool which will encourage you to see and think about the issue through the eyes of someone else; this is called 'others' points of view'.

Apply the exercises below to look at alternative ways to frame the issue that you identified above.

ACTIVITY 5.3

When considering the perceptions of others in healthcare-related issues, we would traditionally consider service users, patients, families, carers, other clinicians or related staff; however, the point of this exercise is to consider the issue from the perspective of another who has no relation to healthcare.

Select one of the following observers (or create one of your own) and think about how this person might describe your issue:

- a seven-year-old child;
- the head of a fast-food chain;
- a football team manager;
- an alien from Mars;
- an events planner;
- an elderly person;
- a politician;
- an airline pilot.

Spend five to ten minutes framing the issue from the new observer's point of view; strive for a number of viewpoints. The purpose is to create connections, generate new ways of seeing the issue or capture perspectives which may be useful to consider later. For example, a football team manager may describe *'How many players will I need and what is the training schedule?'* This might raise thoughts about the people who need to be involved and how a training programme may help.

(Adapted from Maher *et al.*, 2010)

Having spent time on the preparation you should have a clearer framing of the issue and have considered different aspects, gathered any relevant data and spent time on mental reflection, creating different perspectives to consider. All this information will help you articulate your problem or issue to others and will provide the evidence to support the need for innovation.

Imagination

Too many people believe that creativity is a talent with which some people are born and the rest can only envy. This is a negative attitude that is completely mistaken.

(de Bono, 2007)

We will now move to consider the *imagination* phase and look at a few simple ways in which we can increase our creativity to maximise the numbers of ideas we can generate. Few innovations are developed by a single individual without any intervention from others, so you might want to start this phase by making sure you involve the right people with the energy and passion required for maximum creativity. As doctors of tomorrow you will be in a position to enable and lead the staff around you. You will also have the opportunity to be innovative and to support and develop ideas in a team. As Tom Kelley, the Chief Executive of IDEO (an innovation company) and co-author of *The Art of Innovation,* states: *great projects are achieved by great teams* (Kelley and Littleman, 2004).

To allow our imagination and the creative sides of ourselves to take over, and for lots of new ideas to be generated, there needs to be the space both physically and mentally to start the creative process. Sometimes, that means getting away from the office or the busy clinical environment. As Chris Barez-Brown observes, in his book *Shine: How to survive and thrive at work,* people never have the best ideas at their desk; getting away from your usual environment can help and enable you to be more creative (Barez-Brown, 2011). Having a great group of people in a space away from the office does not necessarily mean ideas will just start flowing; often the creative process needs some structure to enable better productive thinking and to help remain focused on one aspect at a time. There are hundreds of tools and techniques for stimulating creative thinking; we will outline two that have been used successfully and which you may like to try.

One well-used technique is that of brainstorming – commonly used, but not always to its full potential. A well-managed brainstorming session can be a great way of generating ideas quickly. Tom Kelley has used the brainstorming technique with his teams, and applies the following five rules (Kelley and Littleman, 2004).

1. Criticism is ruled out – there are no bad ideas and everyone is free to put ideas forward.

2. Go for quantity – aim for at least ten to 20 ideas.

3. Encourage wild ideas – the more far-fetched ideas might be the best ones.

4. Build on the ideas of others – one idea can lead to another and another.

5. Hold one conversation at a time – everyone gets to hear all the ideas.

Other useful tips when conducting a brainstorm to achieve maximum creativity, suggested by Chris Barez-Brown from *Upping Your Elvis* (personal communication, 2011), include the following.

- Use small groups (no more than four people).

- Think of the setting (e.g. sit down on the floor instead of around a table).

- Be clear on the purpose of the brainstorm.

- Use the following matrix to help guide the questions raised in the brainstorm:

  ○ Context – why now? What's the competition?

  ○ Constraints – time, people, money, what am I allowed to do?

  ○ Politics – who is involved with this? Who's on my side? Who's against it?

  ○ Vision of success – if we didn't do anything at all, what would happen?

- Write things down from the middle to the end of the session to capture ideas: 'sit on your pen'; avoid writing the ideas on paper at the start of the brainstorm, otherwise you will lose the essence and energy of what is being said.

- Use drawings to illustrate points raised.

- Complete the brainstorm within five to ten minutes.

Other techniques include association and stimulation as a means of allowing mental connections to be made. One of the leaders in this area of creative thinking is the writer and philosopher Edward de Bono, who introduced the concept of lateral thinking in 1967 because he saw a need to have a way to describe *the sort of thinking that was concerned with changing perceptions and concepts* (de Bono, 1990, 2010). In simple terms, this is the ability to look at things differently, to break out of what de Bono describes as 'mental valleys' or the ways of seeing things in a set way based on what we have been taught. For example, when you think of a hospital ward there will be a certain way of thinking or a mental valley which will bring to mind hospital beds, ward rounds and medicines. To be able to think more creatively, the mind needs to be able to make creative connections to challenge usual taught ways of thinking. Lateral thinking consists of an attitude of mind which is willing to try and look at things in different ways. To help this process and to enable the brain to break away from its usual mental valleys, de Bono devised a number of tools and methods which are described in his numerous books. The following activity is based on a method developed by de Bono which he considers the easiest and the most fun and is formally used by major advertising companies. We would like you to apply your identified issue to Activity 5.4. This method may seem abstract or illogical at first, but it is precisely the seemingly illogical and random nature of the method that serves to tap into lines of creative thinking that might otherwise remain hidden.

ACTIVITY 5.4

Taking your identified issue, challenge or problem, consider how you might come up with ideas to tackle it using the following de Bono random stimulation technique.

Random stimulation is a planned way of encouraging lateral thinking and can be used individually or with groups. This process involves selecting a random word from a dictionary, a pre-prepared word list or a page of text (nouns generally work better). Pictures and images can also be used in a similar way.

To help with this activity we have provided you with a pre-prepared word list.

Start by closing your eyes and placing your finger on a random word from the list.

birth	evolution	technology	management	imagination
cookery	London	computer	children	
family	battle	brain	fuel	health	magic
heart	passenger	mountain	hobbies	rainbow
music	playground	happiness	Walt Disney	
wilderness	seashore	plane	holiday	meadow

Now use the word to start a brainstorming exercise, making new connections between your identified problem or issue and ways in which you could address the problem using the randomly selected word to get ideas flowing – spend about three minutes and at the most five minutes writing down all the ideas that you have generated.

(Adapted from Maher *et al.*, 2010)

Development – taking your idea forward

So now you have an idea – or hopefully a number of ideas – one of which might be the innovative solution you are looking for. So how do you take that idea forward and convince others that this is worth investing time and money in? It is important at this stage that you are able to articulate your idea, problem or need, drawing upon the information that you have gathered from the preparation phase.

For any idea to flourish in a healthcare organisation it needs support from managers and decision makers; bottom-up innovations need top-down effort and prioritisation to succeed (Birkinshaw *et al.*, 2011). It is important therefore that any innovation is grounded in reality and is relevant, appropriate and safe. There are a number of questions that managers, organisations and funders may ask when deciding if an idea is worth taking forward for development; a strong idea will have addressed most of these questions (Table 5.1). The obvious starting point is first to look around to see if someone else has come up with a solution to the problem that you have identified. This horizon-scanning exercise will give you the necessary evidence to support or refute your idea. It may be that during this exercise someone else has solved your problem in a different health sector or industry, in which case your innovation could be about translating your idea into a different setting – your hospital, department or field of practice.

Table 5.1 Questions to ask yourself before taking an idea forward

Question	Consideration
Is it truly innovative?	Has it been done elsewhere before – is there something you can build on to make your idea innovative?
Is there an evidence base?	What evidence or data is there to support the need for the innovation and its impact on the target group? Is there good evidence that similar ideas have worked elsewhere?
Does it fit strategically?	Does your idea meet the objectives and align with the strategic direction of the organisation and the department/service?
What are the benefits?	How does your innovation improve the experience and the outcomes for service users/patients/carers?
What are the risks?	Have all risks been considered and how have they been managed and mitigated against?
Has there been service user/patient/carer involvement?	Have service users/patients/carers been involved in the development of the idea and has there been positive feedback or involvement?
Does it have wider support?	Is there good stakeholder buy-in and support from staff involved?
Will it incur a significant cost?	Is there a cost for the implementation of the innovation? Will it create cost savings whilst maintaining or improving outcomes?
Is the timescale for implementation realistic?	How long will it take to implement the innovation? Have you considered external factors that may impact upon the implementation time, such as new and emerging technologies or new policies?
Is it sustainable?	Is the innovation sustainable over time and does it have a wide impact?
Is it applicable across other areas?	Will the innovation only apply in one area or can it be rolled out across several departments or a whole organisation?

ACTIVITY 5.5

To help you consider your innovative idea, approach or project and to give it a reality check, apply the questions in Table 5.1 to your idea. Consider any gaps and how you might need to make changes to your idea.

We have applied the questions above in a case study example of a service innovation, electronic consultation (e-consultation) in chronic kidney disease, to illustrate these points in more detail.

Case Study

E-consultation using an electronic health record (EHR) has been identified as an innovation with the potential to influence:

- the appropriateness of referrals to secondary care specialist services;
- the overall demand for specialist services in patients with chronic kidney disease (Stoves *et al.*, 2010).

The term 'e-consultation' refers specifically to electronic referral from GP to hospital specialist using the patient's shared EHR. The GP shares the primary care EHR with the hospital specialist after first obtaining verbal patient consent. GPs can use criteria agreed in local guidelines to request advice or question the need for hospital outpatient clinic review. The hospital specialist is able to open the patient's primary care EHR and view important clinical information (e.g. comorbidities, medication history and test results). A decision is then made about where and how the patient's care should be managed. E-consultation allows an electronic opinion about a patient's condition to take place between the specialist and the GP in a timely manner in the context of a collaborative care framework.

We have applied the questions raised by the case study, and relevant to taking an innovation forward, to this service innovation in Table 5.2.

Table 5.2 Questions relevant to taking an innovation forward

Question	Consideration
Is it truly innovative?	Yes. Evidence of e-consultation is limited to our study in Bradford and one other UK study, but the latter was an evaluation of e-mail triage in neurology but not within the context of a shared electronic health record (EHR). Evidence of e-referrals in the USA is promising, but there are substantial gaps in our knowledge about the effectiveness and cost-effectiveness of using e-consultation via an EHR. Evidence is also lacking about the impact upon the patient's experience and population health outcomes.
Is there an evidence base?	Yes. Many inappropriate outpatient referrals for patients with chronic kidney disease can be avoided by measures to improve consultation between primary and secondary care. This requires a GP to seek specialist advice from the renal specialist on patient interventions and for the renal specialist to advise and support GPs as to whether a patient needs referral. This can be managed in primary care with specialist support, or can be managed in primary care alone. Evidence from research in Bradford demonstrated that inappropriate referrals to the renal service were a problem. When GPs were requesting clinic review by letter (traditional method), only 56 per cent of referrals were appropriate according to local criteria (71 per cent and 52 per cent for implementation and non-implementation practices respectively), but 98 per cent of these were accepted for hospital clinic review. By contrast, when using the new service innovation, 90 per cent of e-consultations that questioned the need for clinic review were appropriate, and clinic assessment was recommended in only 27 per cent of cases.
Does it fit strategically?	E-consultation is an example of clinically led, locally negotiated innovation, focused on quality but with the potential to be cost-effective, that is consistent with early indications of the policy direction being set by the UK coalition government.
What are the benefits?	GPs can learn how to manage current patients more effectively and future patients with the same condition as a result of the direct collaboration with hospital specialists which e-consultation affords.
	Support for personalised care: e-consultation supports the health needs of patients/carers by ensuring that their main care-provider can access specialist advice from secondary care consultants, providing a more seamless pathway for the patient and carer.
	Support for 'care closer to home': e-consultation is particularly convenient for patients and carers who either live some distance from an acute hospital or who have difficulty travelling to or from their hospital. Improve access to specialist care through shorter waits and reduced delays (more traditional information flows between consultant and GP add to the patient wait). Individual cases can be prioritised by urgency much more simply than waiting list. Reduce the risk associated with communications (lost letters or faxed referral notes), which are potential threats to patient safety.
What are	GPs would need to be educated on how to use the EHR (in our case Systm One – a centralised IT system allowing a patient's EHR to be shared between

the risks?	primary and secondary care) for e-consultation with a renal specialist. Hospital specialists will also have to learn how to use a primary care EHR – a training programme has been developed and tested in our previous study. Some GPs may be reluctant to change their current practice – we aim to identify those practices that are more or less likely to adopt e-consultation. Not all GP practices in Bradford use Systm One – wider-scale roll out of Systm One is underway. The costs of the service and financial rewards for participating may need clarifying for some GPs and renal specialists – a local tariff has been agreed. Costs and tariffs are both a risk and driver, with the tariff (£23) a very small fee for the effort involved by the specialist team. Acute trusts may have perverse incentives through payment by results to welcome inappropriate referrals.
Has there been service user/ patient/carer involvement?	Yes, GPs and hospital specialists (the users of the service) are fully engaged in the project. Patients have been consulted in the development of the service.
Does it have wider support?	Yes. The e-consultation project is supported by local commissioners, the acute trust and the strategic health authority.
Will it incur a significant cost?	At the time of study, the local tariff for a nephrology outpatient appointment was £237, with follow-up at £117. Our study showed approximately 306 of 376 patients seen in the outpatients clinic (cost £72,522) could have been managed in primary care with the right level of consultant support and guidance. Even if a local e-consult tariff was set at double the non-face-to-face tariff (currently £23), a saving of £58,446 could have been made. The facility for enabling e-consultation within the patient's EHR is readily available, with minimal costs required to enable hospital specialists' access to and training for this facility.
Is the timescale for implementation realistic?	The innovation was initially piloted within chronic kidney disease in 17 early-adopter practices within Bradford (2007–2008), and has since been rolled out to include all practices within Bradford. Regional innovation funding was secured in 2010 to spread this innovation to other specialties, and this work continues with a number of specialties on board. The implementation toolkit which is being produced as an output of this work will speed up implementation, along with software changes made by the EHR developer.
Is it sustainable?	This innovation is sustainable, as the infrastructure (EHR) is in place and is easily modified to support this service innovation. The project also has the support of hospital specialists as a novel means of providing care and as an alternative to hospital outpatient appointments. The training materials (toolkit) developed in our earlier work support the implementation of e-consultation. This service has the ability to impact upon the care of a large number of patients, particularly those with long-term conditions.
Is it applicable across other areas?	This innovation can be rolled out across many specialties, and in our district is already planned for diabetes, rheumatology and cardiology.

Action

To make your idea a reality, you will need to test and implement your idea in practice. This could be by developing a prototype or testing a new way of working. It is important to keep a record of and document the approach you take. Although the implementation of an innovation is beyond the remit of this chapter, you may find the PDSA (plan, do, study, act) cycle a useful approach. You can find out more about this in the next chapter.

Chapter summary

Innovation in healthcare is vital if we want to improve outcomes and services for patients as well as to keep pace with the ever-changing environment in which we live and work. As a doctor of tomorrow you have a crucial role to play in this process, both as a senior clinician and as a reflective practitioner. You will likely lead change for the benefit of patients and as a leader be required to support others to think creatively about the challenges they face and the solutions they could create. In this chapter, we have argued that innovation is your business and indeed the business of every healthcare professional. We have outlined the different types of innovation and described the qualities of successful innovators which you may want to adopt to enable you to be more creative and open to new ideas and concepts.

Being a creative and innovative practitioner is challenging, and as Stephen Lundin (2008) describes, requires overcoming four basic challenges:

1. distractions (doubts and fears accumulated over a lifetime);
2. normal (we develop standard ways of doing things and we need to get outside these norms);
3. failure (most of us try to avoid failure, but we must understand and embrace failure so as to learn from our mistakes);
4. leadership (this plays a vital role in the innovation process in an organisation; leaders need to nurture, develop and support individuals).

Creativity and the desire to do things differently are immensely exciting, interesting and, most importantly, fun, as de Bono points out: *Without creativity there is only repetition and routine* (de Bono, 2007).

The tools and techniques that we have described in this chapter will help equip you to become a creative thinker and promote creative thinking within your clinical team. They will also guide you in ways to take your innovation forward, ensuring that you are ready for the key questions that your consultant, manager, chief executive or funder will ask about your innovation.

> With all that in mind it is always worth remembering the following whilst carrying out your daily procedures, tasks and interventions:
>
> *There's a way to do it better — find it.*
>
> (Thomas Edison)

GOING FURTHER

We have listed a number of websites, books and journals which we personally have used and consider essential reading for those interested in innovation and creativity. The organisations and authors are either at the forefront of modern thinking on innovation or have provided the underpinning theories and models which are still in use today.

The following three websites provide a wealth of information on innovation and further information on tools, techniques and additional resources.

NHS Institute for Innovation and Improvement: **www.institute.nhs.uk**.

The Young Foundation: **www.youngfoundation.org.uk**.

National Endowment for Science, Technology and the Arts: **www.nesta.org.uk**.

Harvard Business Review can be accessed at **www.hbr.org/**. This site provides a range of articles and publications on a wide range of issues relating to innovation.

There are many publications on innovation but there are two authors whose work forms the basis of so many of the models and the thinking on innovation that it is worth exploring their work further. References can be found in the reference list.

Edward de Bono is one of the leading authorities on creative thinking and has published over 70 books. A good starting point is *How to Have Creative Ideas,* which details 62 exercises that you can use yourself or with teams (de Bono, 2007).

Paul Plsek is an internationally recognised consultant on improvement and innovation in complex organisations and has joined with the NHS Institute for Innovation and Improvement to produce a number of publications on innovations and thinking differently. His website **www.directedcreativity.com** outlines much of the work on the directed creativity cycle described in this chapter. His book *Creativity, Innovation and Quality* takes the reader through this from first principle to application (Plsek, 1997).

chapter 6

How to Innovate in Multiprofessional Teams

Beverley Slater and John Bibby

Achieving your medical degree

This chapter will help you to begin to meet the following requirements of *Tomorrow's Doctors* (General Medical Council, 2009a).

Outcome 3 – The doctor as a professional

22. Learn and work effectively within a multiprofessional team:

    (a) Understand and respect the roles and expertise of health and social care professionals in the context of working and learning as a multi-professional team.
    (b) Understand the contribution that effective interdisciplinary team working makes to the delivery of safe and high-quality care.
    (c) Work with colleagues in ways that best serve the interests of patients, passing on information and handing over care, demonstrating flexibility, adaptability and a problem-solving approach.
    (d) Demonstrate ability to build team capacity and positive working relation-ships and undertake various team roles including leadership and the ability to accept leadership by others.

23. Protect patients and improve care:

    (a) Place patients' needs and safety at the centre of the care process.
    (b) Deal effectively with uncertainty and change.
    (d) Promote, monitor and maintain health and safety in the clinical setting, understanding how errors can happen in practice, applying the principles of quality assurance, clinical governance and risk management to medical practice, and understanding responsibilities within the current systems for raising concerns about safety and quality.
    (e) Understand and have experience of the principles and methods of improve-ment, including audit, adverse incident reporting and quality improvement, and how to use the results of audit to improve practice.

Chapter overview

Healthcare professionals work in teams. Teams are both a source of, and a solution to, risks to patient safety. This chapter makes the case for innovating in teams to improve the safety of patients and shows you how to do this. Well-tested improvement tools and case study examples are presented to indicate what resources are available and to illustrate what teams have already achieved by tackling some of the most difficult and pervasive problems in healthcare.

After reading this chapter you will be able to describe the contribution of multi-professional teams working to the delivery of safe care, and will understand the danger of harm from communication problems between healthcare professionals. You will be able to list some of the common tools that are used to support effective teamwork and communication and you will know some of the techniques that have been used to introduce these tools into practice.

Introduction

Having considered in the previous chapter how to be an innovative practitioner, we will now discuss how you can innovate as part of the whole multiprofessional team to improve the safety of the patients in your care.

The majority of all healthcare is delivered in teams, and the vast majority of those teams are multiprofessional. As a doctor you have a specific role to diagnose and treat illness but you will also be working alongside colleagues from a range of professional groups, each contributing to the care that patients need.

As well as the immediate team you work with on a daily basis, the complex nature of healthcare means that there are other levels of team-working in the NHS. For example, where patients need round-the-clock care, there is a sense in which you need to work as a team with those colleagues who are on duty during those hours when you are not. Also, where a patient's care needs stretch between settings (as many care needs do), then there is a need to work as a team across community, hospital and primary care settings. It may not be the norm to consider these staff (many of whom you may never meet) as part of 'your team' but for patients this is clearly the case. Patients assume professionals in the healthcare system routinely communicate and co-ordinate with each other, and are surprised, disappointed and concerned if this is not the case. To fail to communicate properly across a team will put patients' safety at risk, and patients know this (McCullough, 2011; Villette, 2011).

Why innovate in teams?

Healthcare is complex, and the inherent limitations of human performance mean that communication errors between healthcare professionals are inevitable.

Indeed, it is commonly stated that communication failures are a leading contributory cause of patient harm (Sutcliffe *et al.*, 2004; Reader *et al.*, 2007).

Teamwork is equally important in other industries and poor teamwork has led to some of the most well-known transportation disasters, including the 1977 Tenerife airline disaster and the Zeebrugge ferry disaster.

ACTIVITY 6.1

Read about the Zeebrugge ferry disaster at: **en.wikipedia.org/wiki/MS_Herald_ of_Free_Enterprise.**

What were the two most important contributory factors to this incident?

Within healthcare, Leonard and colleagues (2004) make the point that communication and teamwork have not traditionally been the focus for patient safety training; despite the fact that medical care is delivered by multiple team members, safety has traditionally been assumed to be a property of the performance of individual practitioners.

Working as a team around the needs of patients is difficult. But if all of the different healthcare staff are not working in full consultation with their colleagues, then the care will not be focused and co-ordinated around the patient, and patients will be exposed to a risk of gaps, omissions or duplication (Firth-Cozens, 2001a). For example, as it becomes more common to offer 'shared care' between hospital and general practice for people with long-term conditions, so too unfortunately it also becomes more common for patients to be seen without their (monitoring) blood test results being available. This can occur either when the hospital doctor sees patients without the relevant blood results (which were taken in general practice), or, equally, when the GP sees a patient but the relevant blood test results were taken at the hospital.

The good news is that healthcare professionals do not need to work in isolation and that good teamwork is the best guard against the potential fragmentation of care (Leonard *et al.*, 2004; Firth-Cozens, 2001a). Moreover, not only does good teamwork play a major role in creating safer patient care, it is also associated with reduced stress levels. For example, newly qualified UK junior doctors who appreciated that they were part of a multidisciplinary team (as opposed to being bottom of a medical hierarchy) had far lower stress levels that those who did not (Firth-Cozens, 2001b).

There are innovation techniques that can help you to use the resources of the whole multiprofessional team, drawing on the insight and specialist knowledge of colleagues to design, adapt and improve care processes for patients. In addition, teams are able to draw on a range of communication methods and aids which have been developed over recent years; their judicious use in regular practice can support teams to communicate effectively (Leonard *et al.*, 2004).

Not only will this improve the care you offer to patients but it will also help to develop the robust team culture that is necessary to support new members of staff and help them to practise more safely. The prize we are seeking here is to make the whole team better than the sum of its parts. By working together there are opportunities to deliver safer care for patients, and a more rewarding and less stressful working environment for staff.

ACTIVITY 6.2

Consider your current (or most recent) placement in a healthcare setting. Consider the ways in which you worked as a team with other health professionals, and whether you think there was a culture of effective multiprofessional team-working. For example, was there a regular team meeting? Were the relationships between the doctors, nurses and other professional groups easy or fraught?

Thinking about how you keep patients safe during healthcare:

- What are the two most obvious benefits of being part of a team?
- What are two challenges of being part of a team?
- How would you address these?

Now discuss your answers with a colleague and compare your experiences of team-working.

Common issues

There are many different types of multiprofessional teams within healthcare but some core patient safety issues affect all. This is clearly shown in the patient safety issues chosen by multiprofessional teams participating in the *Training and Action for Patient Safety* (TAPS) programme (Slater *et al.*, 2012). Since 2010 we have worked with over 50 multiprofessional teams from the whole range of healthcare contexts, including hospital care, mental health care, primary medical care and nursing homes, each of which has been seeking to improve the safety of patient care in its area. Teams were asked to identify up to three current patient safety concerns and then choose which to address. Figure 6.1 presents an overview of the types of patient safety issues that the teams chose to focus on. Across all settings, communication issues (including handover between shifts and patient transfer between locations) were the most common category.

However, most of the patient safety issues in the other categories would also involve an element of communication in addressing the problem. Examples include medicines reconciliation when a patient moves between different care settings, implementing good nutritional assessment practices in hospital and developing good practices in escalating the response to a deteriorating patient. Although communication is a common factor in many of these issues, getting people to understand

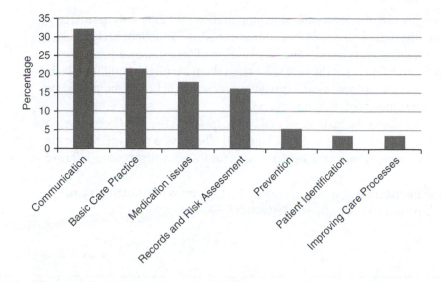

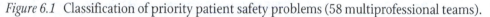

Figure 6.1 Classification of priority patient safety problems (58 multiprofessional teams).

and believe that communication is one of the most potent threats to patient safety can be a challenge in itself.

Common solutions

The common patient safety issues (such as communication, medication management and execution of basic care practices) are generally well recognised within health services, but so too are some of the solutions. Many of these have their impact through supporting effective team communication. Common solutions include the following.

Checklists

Checklists are a common feature of the healthcare environment, serving both as a memory aid and a potential audit tool to assess compliance. Checklists are used when introducing a standardised 'care bundle' for a particular patient group undergoing particular treatment. The most famous patient safety checklist is the World Health Organization (WHO) surgical safety checklist, which has been associated with one-third reduction in postoperative complications and deaths in hospitals located across diverse geographic and economic environments (Haynes *et al.*, 2011).

Structured communication tools

What we *want* to communicate and what is *actually* communicated often differ. Fortunately there are several effective tools to assist with structured communication.

These tools are useful in most clinical communications but especially in emergency situations. The most widely used tool is known as SBAR (Situation, Background, Assessment, Recommendation). The SBAR tool provides a framework for communication between members of the healthcare team about a patient's condition. It allows for an easy and focused way to set expectations for *what* will be communicated and *how* between members of the team.

Figure 6.2 shows the basic SBAR tool and adaptations that have been developed (another one, SBARR, was covered in Chapter 2). The version used will be a matter of local preference. In each case the elements of the framework should be followed in order.

For an interactive video demonstrating this tool, see **www.nottingham. ac.uk/nmp/sonet/rlos/patientsafety/sbar/**.

Basic SBAR	ISBAR (when professionals do not know each other)
Situation 'I am concerned about…'	**Introduction** 'I am….; my role is…'
Background 'Patient history is…'	**Situation** 'I am concerned about…'
Assessment Vital signs/clinical impression	**Background** 'Patient history is…'
Recommendation 'I need from you…'	**Assessment** Vital signs/clinical impression
	Recommendation 'I need from you…'
ISBARR (to include review of decision reached)	**ISBARD** (to explicitly refer to decision reached)
Introduction 'I am….; my role is…'	**Introduction** 'I am….; my role is…'
Situation 'I am concerned about…'	**Situation** 'I am concerned about…'
Background 'Patient history is…'	**Background** 'Patient history is…'
Assessment Vital signs/clinical impression	**Assessment** Vital signs/clinical impression
Recommendation 'I need from you…'	**Recommendation** 'I need from you…'
Review Clarify orders, expectations and time frame	**Decision** 'Hence, what we have decided is…'

Figure 6.2 SBAR (Situation, Background, Assessment and Recommendation) and adaptations.

Situational awareness training

Situational awareness is an important concept for avoiding error or mitigating potential harm in safety-critical tasks. Training resources, using video or simulation, aim to improve situational awareness of the individual health professional, but may also include recognition of the value of the team contribution through 'distributed' situational awareness.

Crew resource management, and other training to enhance team-working

The term 'crew resource management' has been borrowed from the airline industry and is increasingly applied in healthcare settings. CRM refers to non-technical skills, such as situation awareness, decision-making and teamwork, that team members ('crew') need to deliver their tasks safely and effectively. The message is that technical skills alone are not sufficient to ensure safety, whether in the airline industry or in healthcare. There have been calls for CRM training to be integrated into undergraduate curricula (Flin and Patey, 2009) to help doctors and other staff to be alert to the importance of non-technical skills, and to increase the acceptance of this training as an ongoing part of multiprofessional team practice.

Design solutions

Some patient safety problems arise from a poorly designed interface between a medical device and the medical staff using that device. In Chapter 4 Peter Gardner describes the principles behind good design. Although primarily derived for use with complex technologies, these principles can be applied to more simple technologies used and adapted in everyday practice, including the charts and checklists used by staff. When designing aids to help prompt and sustain safe practice, it is important for teams to remember to review against the principles of good design and, crucially, include staff users at every stage of the design process.

Innovation within teams means understanding the patient safety issue or gap, and then identifying a solution and bringing it into practice. By bringing a solution into practice the team will adapt it to make sense within their particular environment, perhaps adding a new feature or delivering in a new way. In this way teams produce something innovative within their own practice that, in turn, may be of interest for other teams to consider and adapt to their own context.

Innovation in teams – the basics

Understanding patient safety

Before being able to innovate to improve patient safety, the team members you work with will need to be able to identify patient safety issues within the professional environment. This will build on patient safety education and training that should be consolidated throughout one's professional life, through prequalification and postgraduate training and continuing professional development. Some of this training may have been multiprofessional, for example through simulation training.

Although training for all professional groups together may be the ideal, it is nevertheless worth recognising that some of your older colleagues may never have received training in patient safety principles and ways of understanding error. This could potentially cause difficulties if colleagues feel uncomfortable or defensive when considering potential sources of error in the practice environment. It may be worth managers within your team environment being aware of online courses that offer an introduction to patient safety to members of staff who may have missed out on some of the basic concepts.

Leadership and governance

Innovation in teams requires some degree of leadership. Innovation is unlikely to emerge without some co-ordination, consolidation and the drive to make improvements. Does this need to come from the most senior person in the team? Surprisingly, the answer is 'no'. Anyone within a team can step forward for this role, using a model of participatory leadership. The qualities needed to lead a team where innovation can flourish are firstly, a passion for improving the identified issue and secondly, a willingness to drive the work forward by facilitating colleagues' contributions. Juniors are in a good position to be participatory leaders of improvement work. As a new member of a team with 'fresh eyes', a medical student or junior doctor is often better able to see cracks in team-working or culture and to adopt new ideas and ways.

Many juniors feel that to be a leader you need to be in a position of authority, such as a consultant or senior doctor. This could not be further from the truth. Leadership theories have developed from the early 'heroic' models prior to 1990 through the 'trait' models, stressing situational and environmental factors, to more recent integration, engaging or participatory models, stressing interpersonal skills (Alimo-Metcalf and Alban-Metcalf, 2002, pp 300–25; McKimm and Forrest, 2011). There is still a role for position 'power leadership' but the ability to improve team-working and culture is largely determined by participatory and collaborative leadership.

Modern healthcare is not an individual activity but is carried out by teams working within systems. The safety and quality of care provided depend upon the performance of the individual, the team and the system. Clinical governance is the process by which health services are held accountable for the safety, quality and effectiveness of clinical care delivered to patients.

Clinical governance is a statutory requirement of all NHS organisations and is achieved by co-ordinating three interlinking strands of work:

1. robust national and local systems and structures that help identify, implement and report on quality improvement;

2. quality improvement work involving healthcare staff, patients and the public;

3. establishing a supportive, inclusive learning culture for improvement.

The original definition from 1998 still holds true:

Clinical governance is a system through which NHS organisations are account-
able for continuously improving the quality of their services and safeguarding high
standards of care by creating an environment in which excellence in clinical care will
flourish.

(Scally and Donaldson, 1998, p61)

Effective leadership will lead to a culture in which good clinical governance
flourishes.

Principles of team improvement

Since 2000 there have been many examples of multiprofessional team-based innovation and improvement across the NHS. There has been increasing consensus on the
requirements for effective improvement work (Kennedy *et al.*, 2009; Health Foundation, 2011). Our experience of working with several hundred teams across the UK
over the past ten years leads us to offer the following key advice to anyone who is
preparing to support innovation and improvement in a work setting.

Get the right team together

This should be a group of four to six people who are interested in improving the service, and who can represent and give feedback to the main front-line staff who know
about this issue.

Agree regular meetings

Regular short meetings are better for making progress than infrequent longer meetings – so, for example, meeting for 15 minutes at 8.30 a.m. every Monday morning is
preferred to a two-hour project meeting every two months.

Seek patient perspectives

The patients' perspective complements the clinicians' perspective on healthcare
and will often provide information that surprises the staff who may work every day
on the unit. Patients may be part of the improvement team or their views sought
through separate consultation. The involvement of a patient perspective will help the
team to check out and confirm priorities and potential impact.

Real-time measurement (or as close as possible)

Real-time measurement of improvement provides feedback to the team that is both
motivating and empowering. This will usually be measurement for improvement
(under the control of the team) rather than measurement for the purpose of demonstrating performance to external agencies.

Innovate/review in small change cycles

An essential approach to intelligent learning from doing is sometimes referred to as the plan–do–study–act (PDSA) approach (see tool 7 below). This should become a way of thinking about change.

Give feedback to the wider team

The small team needs to build in feedback to senior management and to the wider team if the improvement is to be sustainable in the medium to long term.

Innovation in teams – tools and techniques

Once you have a team that is willing to work together to improve patient safety there are a range of tools and techniques to help you identify priorities and start to make a difference.

Identifying your patient safety priorities

Tool 1: Two simple questions

A technique to reveal the knowledge of the team gained through experience, and to engage everyone in understanding what can be improved, is simply to ask the following two questions:

1. *What was our last patient safety issue?*

2. *What will be our next one?*

After taking a minute or two for everyone to think through their response, discuss your answers as a multidisciplinary team. This will help you to pinpoint where you might need to improve patient safety, and to start a healthy discussion between different team members.

Tip

If some of the team members are not used to sharing with each other on an equal basis, you should suggest that people share their answers in pairs before having a wider discussion as a team.

To consider

Could you also consider asking patients about the risks that they see?

Tool 2: Trigger tools

Although asking staff the two simple questions above can be revealing and insightful, the disadvantages are that this is a subjective measure which focuses on rare but memorable events. To obtain a more objective measure of errors in practice, the idea of measuring the incidence of adverse events by assessing case notes has been developed. Case note reviews are objective, focus on outcomes and on the more common adverse events, and have been shown to be reliable over time (Chapter 7). However, since analysing large numbers of case notes is very resource-intensive, a model of case note review using trigger tools has been developed. This involves case reviews that are filtered and targeted, and hence is quicker, cheaper and less wasteful. The Global Trigger Tool (GTT), developed by the Institute for Healthcare Improvement, makes use of 'triggers', or clues, to identify adverse events and is an effective method for measuring the overall level of harm in a healthcare organisation (Classen *et al.*, 2008).

How the GTT works

A defined number (x) of records are selected randomly to be reviewed each month, searching for the presence of predefined 'triggers' that signify a risk of harm. Those records that have the trigger(s) present are then looked at in more detail for the presence of actual harm events (y). The ratio of harm events divided by the number of records analysed (x/y) is the *event rate*. This event rate can be displayed each month on a runchart (see Tool 3 below) to give a visual representation of the organisation's adverse event rate. For a more detailed discussion, watch the video at: **www.insti-tute.nhs.uk/safer_care/safer_care/trigger_tool_portal.html**.

Measures for improvement

Tool 3: The simple runchart

When thinking about improving services, doctors tend to be more familiar with the 'before and after' audit, but far more flexible and powerful is the simple runchart (Perla *et al.*, 2011). The simplest runchart with which you are familiar is the TPR (temperature, pulse and respiration) chart. The key to using runcharts to bring about change is to identify a pragmatic measure that can be assessed daily or weekly and that is an indicator of the issue in question (Figure 6.3). More information about selecting appropriate measures is given in Chapter 7.

Identifying innovations

Tool 4: Fishbone diagram

The fishbone diagram is a graphic tool used to explore and display all the factors that may influence, or cause, a given outcome. Figure 6.4 gives an example of a fishbone diagram constructed by a team starting to explore handover problems at the end of a shift.

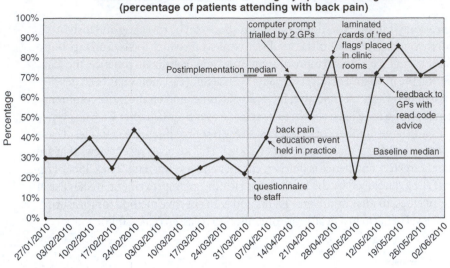

Figure 6.3 A simple annotated runchart.

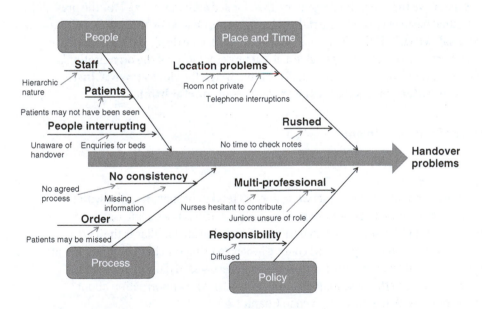

Figure 6.4 Fishbone diagram to understand the causes of poor handover between staff.

Purpose

- to determine root causes of a given effect;

- to illustrate the interaction of many causes rather than a single cause for a given effect;

- to explore systematically an answer to the question 'why?';
- to identify the various sources of variation affecting a given key quality characteristic by systematically sorting and relating those sources to the effect;
- to identify areas where there is a lack of data, or a need to collect data to determine significance of cause.

How to construct a cause-and-effect diagram

1. Agree on a single statement that describes the effect. (You may wish to make it the problem (what is wrong?) or preferably the objective (what would you like to see?).)

2. Write a statement that describes the effect – the key quality characteristic.

3. Set major categories as 'bones' (e.g. policies, procedures, people, methods, materials, equipment, environment).

4. Place brainstorming ideas as branches under the appropriate category. There will be factors and subfactors.

Tool 5: Process map

A process map is a graphical representation of all the major steps of a process. The purpose is to help understand a complete process: Who does what? And why? Done as a team activity, constructing a process map will show relationships between different steps in a process, help to identify the critical stages and problem areas and indicate appropriate data collection points.

How to construct and use a process map

1. Identify the process. Define the start point and finish point for the process to be examined.

2. Describe the *current* process. Chart the whole process (lay out all the steps) from beginning to end. You can use symbols shown below to improve the clarity of your flow chart, but sticky notes are simpler and more effective.

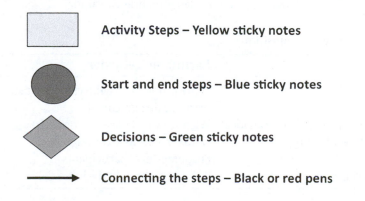

Activity Steps – Yellow sticky notes

Start and end steps – Blue sticky notes

Decisions – Green sticky notes

Connecting the steps – Black or red pens

3. (Optional) Chart the *ideal* process. Try to identify the easiest and most efficient way to go from the 'start block'. While this step isn't absolutely necessary, it does make it easier to do the next step.

4. Search for improvement opportunities. Identify all the areas that hinder your process or add little or no value. If you did the previous (optional) step, examine all areas that differ from your ideal process and question why they exist.

5. Update your map. Build a new process map that corrects the problems you identified in the previous step.

Analysing your process map

Once the process is agreed, it is worth analysing the process map for any further opportunities for improvement.

- Rework loops. Are there rework loops where activities are repeated due to failures in the process? Could these be eliminated? What is the cost of the rework loop in terms of number of steps, lost time and resources? Does the rework loop prevent the problem recurring?

- Delay/wait. Are there pauses or times when waiting is involved (delay/wait symbols)? Does this cause further complexity? How can it be reduced or how can we reduce its impact?

- Activity. Is the activity necessary? What is the value of the activity relative to its cost? How have errors been prevented in this activity?

Tool 6: Brainstorm

Brainstorming is a group decision-making technique designed to generate a large number of creative ideas through an interactive process. The purpose is to create a lot of ideas in a short time from all participants, without criticism or judgment, and which then can be evaluated in a later stage. An effective way has been described in Chapter 5. In many health service teams a pragmatic way of doing this is to follow well-defined guidelines to break down barriers between existing and new teams. We suggest you look again at pages 89–90 to remind yourself of Tom Kelley's five rules for brainstorming (Kelley and Littleman, 2004), and of Chris Barez-Brown's (2011) tips for maximising creativity.

Table 6.1 will help to consolidate your knowledge on brainstorming.

Table 6.1 How to conduct a brainstorm

Participants	Facilitator/recorder
One idea in turn	Write problem on a flip chart for all to see and gain agreement
Pass if the participant doesn't have an idea	Write down all ideas as presented
Lots of ideas and freewheeling	Number each item for reference
Laughter is OK	Encourage non-participants
No criticism, no ridicule	Encourage through the lulls

Testing and action learning

Tool 7: Small change cycles

The small change cycle, sometimes known as the PDSA cycle, is a tried and tested approach to developing and implementing change. The stages of the PDSA cycle are as follows:

P: Plan. This stage involves identifying the changes that will be made, setting objectives, making predictions and planning how to measure the outcomes. It will also involve identifying what will be done, roles and responsibilities and timescales. The results of the PDSA cycle are dependent on the quality of the plan.

D: Do. This is the stage where the plan is put into action. Data for monitoring and measuring the changes will be collected and observations recorded.

S: Study. At this stage, progression is reviewed and reflected on. The collected data will be analysed and compared with predictions. Any ideas for improvements to the cycle should be raised.

A: Act. This stage involves looking forward to the next stage. It may be that the cycle should be run again with improvements made, or further cycles should be created to develop the changes.

PDSA cycles are small-scale, reflective tests used to try out ideas for improvement. They can be repeated and built upon to achieve more significant changes. Use it to break down a change into manageable chunks that you can implement with minimal disruption.

Advantages of PDSA cycles

- uncomplicated, yet highly effective;
- small changes mean small risks and small expenditure;
- changes are quick and immediately evident;
- team members can provide input so strategies can be tailored to their needs;
- changes can be focused at the operational level around your team's needs.

The cycles should be small and simple. In this way, getting started is easy, and you can move quickly through each stage and apply the learning quickly. It also reduces risk, as anything that goes wrong will not have a large impact. Running a few successive cycles will build on learning and allow effective, easily accomplishable and proven changes to the system.

In order to identify ideas to test using PDSA cycles, you need to take time to consider the following questions:

- What are we trying to accomplish?
- How will we know that a change is an improvement?
- What changes can we make that will result in improvement?

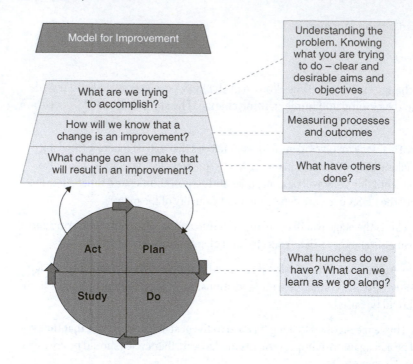

Figure 6.5 Using PDSA (plan, do, study, act) cycles. (Adapted with permission from Langley *et al.*, 2009.)

The ideas that emerge can then be tested using PDSA cycles (Figure 6.5).

Presenting information

Tool 8: Keep it simple, visual and current

Visual information, regularly updated and pinned up in an area the team regularly passes (staff room or equivalent) is the best way to communicate progress, and keep a team involved and interested. Charts are most effective when they plot just one dimension, so that anyone reading them can immediately identify what is going on with the project. If the team have been involved in choosing what is tracked then they are more likely to be engaged in learning from the results.

Consolidation, sustainability and spread

Tool 9: The NHS sustainability tool

A perennial problem with quality improvement processes in the NHS is that, even with projects that show an improvement, the majority are not sustained. The factors that determine the likelihood of sustainability have been characterised under three domains: process, staff and organisation.

Process

- benefits beyond helping patients – making the job easier;
- credibility of benefits – obvious, evidence-based, believed;
- adaptability of improved process – continuous improvement;
- effectiveness of system to monitor process – communication of results.

Staff

- staff involvement and training to sustain process;
- staff attitudes towards sustaining change – involvement and empowerment;
- senior leadership engagement – responsibility and advice;
- clinical leadership engagement – responsibility and advice.

Organisation

- fit with organisation's strategic aims and culture – history of improvement, consistency of improvement goals with strategic aims;
- infrastructure for sustainability – staff, facilities and equipment.

The NHS sustainability tool has been developed and helps teams to assess the strength of the above factors. This tool is available from the NHS Institute for Innovation and Improvement website (**www.institute.nhs.uk**). This tool is most usefully applied to any proposed improvement before embarking on a large amount of work. Depending on the outcome of using the tool it may be necessary for the team to make some internal adjustments even before they start their project.

An alternative tool is the Team Climate Inventory (Anderson and West, 1998), which was developed to measure the climate for innovation within teams at work.

Learning from other teams

Tool 10: Peer review

If you are undertaking improvement work as part of a structured programme there may be an opportunity to undertake peer review with another team or teams. Unlike the site visit (Tool 11 below), this method works well with a team working in a completely different area of healthcare to your own. We run peer review sessions at all our team improvement events. The secret of this technique is that the other team is an outsider to your situation, so the questions they ask you may uncover something that insiders like yourself never think to question. Teams working in different areas of healthcare do not consider themselves to be in competition with each other and so, in our experience of running this type of session, participants will usually be honest, supportive and interested.

Elements of a peer review session (30–40 minutes)

- Step 1: Introductions (five to seven minutes).
- Step 2: Team A briefly describe their safety issue and why it is a priority (five to seven minutes).
- Step 3: Team B ask questions of clarification (two to three minutes).
- Step 4: Team B ask questions to stimulate thinking (not aiming to give advice) (five to seven minutes).
- Step 5: Conclude discussion of team A. Repeat steps two to four for team B (15 minutes).

Tool 11: The site visit

As a medical student, and later on as a junior doctor, you have the opportunity to visit many different healthcare facilities. This is a natural opportunity for you to observe and understand how different teams and organisations are tackling the same patient safety issues and the innovations that they have developed. Established teams who do not rotate do not have this opportunity built into their work pattern and so may need to consider a formal 'site visit' to get the equivalent experience and understanding. As someone with recent experience of other units, your advice might be sought on other units that have developed interesting innovative approaches. Formal site visits between teams can be very beneficial. The other team is likely to be flattered that you want to visit and your team may gain some ideas – or alternatively realise that you already have ideas within your own team and be motivated to develop these.

Innovation in teams – bringing it all together

The following case studies show how teams in different settings have delivered patient safety improvements.

ACTIVITY 6.3

Read through the three case studies in this chapter, all taken from the TAPS programme. Consider the one that is closest to your experience so far:

- From your experience, do you recognise the patient safety issue identified by the team?
- Is this a current issue in your area of practice?
- What do you think of the solutions generated by the team?
- How would you introduce these ideas to teams that you are a member of?
- Could these ideas be adapted and adopted by those teams?

Case Study 1: Medicines reconciliation in general practice: improving communication about medication changes for patients with a dosette box

Identifying patient safety priorities

A GP met with a GP registrar and a receptionist to discuss patient safety concerns in the practice. They were aware of several errors that had occurred when patients with dosette boxes had a medication changed. (Note: A dosette box is a packaging system to help patients take the right tablets at the right time, often provided for patients who are elderly or confused.)

Measures for improvement

The team recorded the number of queries relating to dosette boxes from the pharmacy to the general practice. Retrospective data were available from the local pharmacist.

Identifying innovations

There was no system to communicate clearly when a change was needed to one of the medications in a dosette box, and this was leading to many queries between pharmacy and GP practice. The team devised a proforma to communicate these changes.

Testing and action learning

This was introduced and then, in the light of experience and consultation, revised.

Presenting information

Figure 6.6 (overleaf) shows how information about dosette boxes can be presented in a graph.

Consolidation, sustainability and spread

The revised proforma has been in continuous use for more than a year. Other general practices have heard about it and are using it.

Learning with other teams

This team benefited from discussing the innovations being developed by other general practice teams on the TAPS programme.

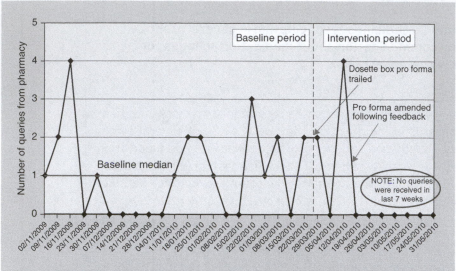

Figure 6.6 Dosette box queries received from pharmacy.

Case Study 2: Reducing episodes of violence and aggression in a mental health ward

Identifying patient safety priorities

A small team consisting of two mental health nurses, a junior doctor, occupational therapist, pharmacist and the audit and knowledge manager identified self-harm by patients on the ward as a problem that was having a negative effect on both patients and staff.

Measures for improvement

The team collected the number of incidents of self-harm.

Identifying innovations

The smaller team worked through the issue using the fishbone methodology (tool 4 above) and then involved the whole team using six de Bono hats* to pull together ideas for interventions. The team decided to involve patients in their care from the start, place less emphasis on one-to-one interventions (which controlled patients but did not

---

* This is a creativity tool where members of the group are encouraged to see problems and solutions in new ways according to the colour of the hat they are wearing. There are six differently coloured hats, each representing a different perspective: white, objective; red, intuitive; black, negative; yellow, positive; green, creative; and blue, process.

offer anything to solve the problem), identified alternative strategies (such as ice cubes, stress balls, elastic bands, going for walks) and put up a poster on the wall reminding everyone of the alternative strategies.

Testing and action learning

The interventions were introduced and the impact on the weekly incidents of self-harm was noticeable.

Presenting information

The information was presented in the form of a graph (Figure 6.7).

Consolidation, sustainability and spread

Despite being busy, the team has embraced the experience of learning together and have seen their ideas come into practice. They are planning to use a similar approach with a smaller then wider team to look at the approach to missing persons.

Learning with other teams

This team benefited by learning from teams tackling issues in other settings, including general practice and hospital wards.

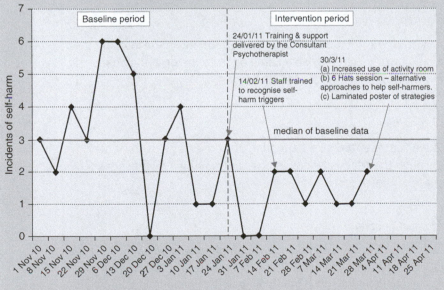

Figure 6.7 The number of incidents of self-harm occurring on the ward.

Case Study 3: Improving venous thromboembolism risk assessment in the hospital medical admissions ward

Identifying patient safety priorities

Venous thromboembolism (VTE) is a preventable harm that occurs if patients are not assessed and then treated with an appropriate prophylactic. This was a priority for the hospital, and this team from the preassessment clinic used the TAPS programme to understand why it was not happening within their unit and to address this.

Measures for improvement

The measures for improvement included the percentage of admitted patients being assessed for VTE risk.

Identifying innovations

The team, comprising consultants, junior doctors, pharmacist, ward manager and clinical educator, used the fishbone diagram (tool 4) to identify the different barriers that prevent completion of the VTE assessment and then to identify possible interventions. Ideas included using a 'safety cross', an admission bookmark on the notes, a poster for medical staff, a revised poster showing financial implications, e-mail from the clinical director and introducing electronic pens.

Testing and action learning

A new intervention was introduced each week, building on the last one. If one idea didn't work then the team came back to the drawing board to consider others.

Presenting information

The results were presented as a daily plot of percentage of patients admitted through the Medical Admissions Unit having a VTE assessment completed (Figure 6.8).

Consolidation, sustainability and spread

The team has maintained 95–98 per cent compliance rate and it has now become part of the way of work. The project manager is spreading this way of working in her hospital by working with clinicians who know TAPS to use it within their own peer groups.

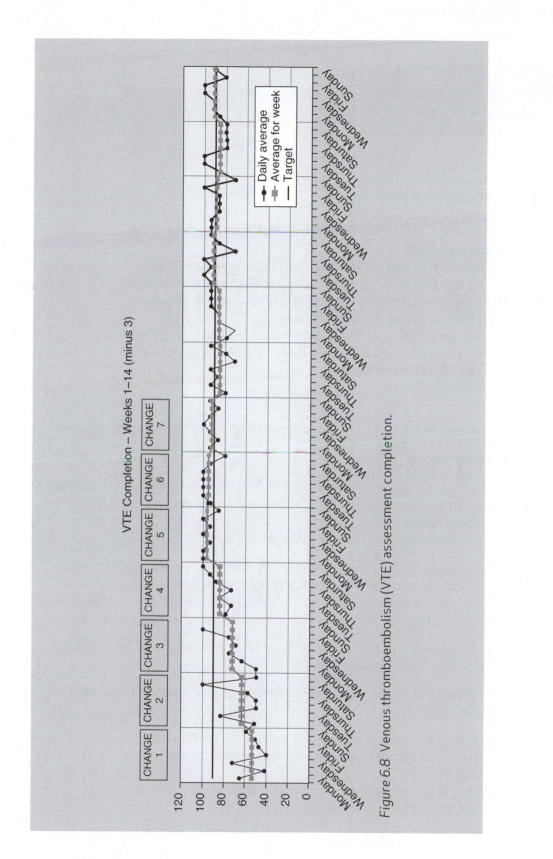

Figure 6.8 Venous thromboembolism (VTE) assessment completion.

> *Learning with other teams*
>
> This team benefited from learning from other teams within their own hospital tackling other patient safety issues.

Finally, if you do only one thing

The final message at the conclusion of this chapter is that if you are able to do only one thing, please make it this.

Do encourage any team that you are working in to have regular meetings to reflect on and discuss the care you are giving, if possible allowing time at the beginning or end of those meetings where people can be allowed to suggest new ways of tackling the problems and issues that inevitably arise.

If, in addition, you are able to have some learning and continuing professional education together as a multidisciplinary team, then your path towards safer and more effective care will be enhanced.

Chapter summary

Most of us will not practise in isolation but will be delivering care as part of a team. Working in teams can help or hinder patient safety. As patient care becomes more complex, the number of teams involved in a patient's care increase. Hence a focus on the team is an integral part of improving patient safety.

This chapter has encouraged you to reflect on how the teams you work in function and to evaluate your contribution to the team. Various tools to evaluate the team's likelihood of success in improving patient safety have been introduced along with tools and techniques to help you and the team bring about improvements in patient safety.

The use of the model for improvement with the associated use of small change cycles (PDSAs) is strongly advocated.

The key elements of increasing the effectiveness of your involvement in patient safety are as follows.

1. Be clear what you are trying to achieve and use the tools to bring this about.
2. Understand how you will measure any improvement, especially making use of runcharts.
3. Test changes out before making wholesale change.
4. Communicate, communicate, communicate.

GOING FURTHER

Perla, RJ, Provost, LP and Murray, SK (2011) The run chart: a simple analytical tool for learning from variation in healthcare processes. *BMJ Quality and Safety in Health Care*, 20: 46–51.
Measurement for improvement is important for motivating teams. This article by Perla and colleagues is a clear, simple and practical explanation of runcharts.

Situational Awareness Vital Insights (SAVI) training videos, which are particularly useful for new clinical staff, can be accessed at **www.training-pod.com/savi**.

Weaver, S, Rosen, M, Salas, E, Baum, K and King, H (2010) Integrating the science of team training: guidelines for continuing education. *Journal of Continuing Education in the Health Professions*, 30(4): 208–20.
A fuller description of the teamwork competencies that can be enhanced through continuing professional development training is included in this article.

The TAPS website (**www.nhstaps.org**) is useful to help you and your team on your patient safety improvement journey.

chapter 7

How Safe Are You? Measurement for **Patient Safety**

Rebecca Lawton and Gerry Armitage

Achieving your medical degree

This chapter will help you to begin to meet the following requirements of *Tomorrow's Doctors* (General Medical Council, 2009a).

Outcome 2: The doctor as scholar and scientist

The graduate will be able to:

11 (c) Describe measurement methods relevant to the improvement of clinical effectiveness and care.

Outcome 3: The doctor as professional

The graduate will be able to:

23 (e) Understand and have experience of the principles and methods of improvement, including audit, adverse incident reporting and quality improvement, and how to use the results of audit to improve practice.

Moreover, this chapter aligns with the explicit focus on patient safety (Domain 1 of *Tomorrow's Doctors*, 2009) and the specific outcomes relating to patient safety in your undergraduate curriculum.

Chapter overview

As a medical student and foundation doctor it is important that you are able to assess how well you are doing (as part of a healthcare system, organisation or team) in patient safety. To do this, effective measurement is necessary. In this chapter we will explain why there is no definitive measure of patient safety, but that appropriate measurement depends on the *definition of patient safety* and the *purpose of the measurement*. We present different ways of measuring safety and explain their strengths and weaknesses. This will help you to understand which measure is appropriate to the question you want to answer, as well as how measurement can help to improve your own and others' clinical practice.

After reading this chapter you will be able to:

• describe what a good measure looks like;
• outline the strengths and weaknesses of different measures of patient safety;
• understand how to measure patient safety depending on circumstances;
• consider how measurement can be used to improve clinical practice.

Introduction: why measure patient safety?

In Chapter 4, you learned about Wayne Jowett, a young man recovering from leukaemia, who went into hospital to be given vincristine and methotrexate. As you know, this routine procedure resulted in disaster. In Chapter 4, Peter Gardner discussed the technical aspects of the case from a human factors perspective. We will now take another look at the case but to illustrate a very different point. The following excerpt is taken from the external inquiry into this event (Toft, 2001):

> At approximately 17.00 hours on Thursday 4th January 2001, Mr Wayne Jowett, a day case patient on Ward E17 at the Queen's Medical Centre Nottingham (QMC), was prepared for an intrathecal (spinal) administration of chemotherapy as part of his medical maintenance programme following successful treatment of leukaemia. After carrying out a lumbar puncture and administering the correct cytotoxic therapy (cytosine) under the supervision of the Specialist Registrar Dr Mulhem, Dr Morton, a Senior House Officer, was passed a second drug by Dr Mulhem to administer to Mr Jowett, which he subsequently did. However, the second drug, vincristine, should never be administered by the intrathecal route because it is almost always fatal. Unfortunately, whilst emergency treatment was provided very quickly in an effort to rectify the error, Mr Jowett died at 8.10 AM on the 2nd February 2001.

Although the formal inquiry provides a very matter-of-fact account of events, the media took quite a different approach, emphasising numerous causes but focusing on the individual culpability of the doctors and what action should be taken against them. Here is an excerpt from a BBC news article at the time:

> Investigators have revealed that a catalogue of blunders led to the death of teenager Wayne Jowett.
>
> Wayne, aged 18, died in February at the Queen's Medical Centre, Nottingham, after a cancer drug was wrongly injected into his spine rather than a vein.
>
> An independent report has criticised staff and procedures at the hospital and another report has highlighted design faults in syringes and drug packaging.
>
> One investigator said the 'entire' staff on the day ward where Wayne was treated had been 'lulled into a false sense of security' and had forgotten that mistakes could be made.
>
> **(news.bbc.co.uk/1/hi/health/1284244.stm)**

ACTIVITY 7.1

Having read the BBC news clip, now consider the first three paragraphs of the *British Medical Journal* piece: 'The criminalisation of fatal medical mistakes' by Jon Holbrook, barrister, published on 13 November 2003, which you can find at **www.bmj.com/content/327/7424/1118.full**.

Discuss with one or two peers whether you agree with the argument put forward in this article.

Much interest in patient safety stems from events of this kind, where attention is commonly and inappropriately focused on the individuals who were closest to the incident. It is unfortunate that our focus when discussing patient safety is so often on negative outcomes, in other words the breakdown of safety. In fact, without a scientific approach that is characterised by valid and transparent measurement, we will continue to struggle in our attempt to move beyond this blame-driven approach and towards a focus on how to improve safety. Ongoing measurement of safety events and clear identification of causes, as well as measurement of compliance with procedures and effectiveness of clinical processes, can help to identify problems with safety before they occur and therefore reduce potential harm to patients and the blame of individual clinicians. Measurement for patient safety actually serves a number of purposes for different stakeholders. These include hospital managers' and external regulators' requirement to monitor safety performance, local health professionals' evaluations of whether a specific change in practice or procedure has improved safety and researchers' desire to understand or test interventions to improve patient safety for the general population. The way in which patient safety is defined and measured depends, at least to some extent, on for what purpose and on whom measurement is being carried out.

In this chapter, we will help you to understand the importance of measurement for improving patient safety and preventing harm. Measurement is a very complex topic area, so here we will focus on the core concepts that are important for you, as a medical student/foundation doctor, to understand in order to meet the standards for professional practice. Therefore we address the following questions in this chapter:

- What is patient safety and what does a good measure look like?
- How do you measure patient safety?
- How can measurement help in my practice?

What is patient safety?

The way something is measured depends on what that 'something' is. For example, in order to decide whether or not an individual is binge drinking you must first have a clear definition of what constitutes binge drinking. So, you must, in this case, decide how many units of alcohol represent a 'binge' and over what time period these units have to be consumed. The NHS definition of binge drinking is consuming eight or more units in a single session for men and six or more for women (**www.nhs.uk/ Livewell/alcohol/Pages/Bingedrinking.aspx**).

Binge drinking might appear an easy concept to define and measure, but even here there is debate. For example, it is difficult to define a clear time period over which excess alcohol is consumed because tolerance and speed of drinking in a session vary from person to person. Moreover, the definition of binge drinking has changed over time, once referring to going on a binge of heavy drinking over a period of several days, but now referring to one uninterrupted session of drinking (Berridge *et al.*, 2009). This demonstrates that measurement is a function of the way in which the concept is defined which, in turn, is heavily influenced by social and economic change.

Let's look at another example in clinical practice. In 2006, the National Institute for Health and Clinical Excellence (p10) defined hypertension as: *when either systolic pressure exceeds 140 mmHg or diastolic blood pressure exceeds 90 mmHg.* However, while this is a relatively straightforward definition of a tangible phenomenon, measurement is not so simple. Several critical factors should also be considered.

- The patient's blood pressure should be measured on both arms with an appropriate width to the cuff.

- Measurement should be taken on more than one occasion.

- The patient's emotional state can affect the result.

In these two cases (alcohol consumption and blood pressure), numerical values provide data about the normal and conversely the abnormal. Yet even here there are difficulties because quantitative measurement is affected by the advancement of science (and hence changes in definition), economic or cost considerations (for example, treating large-scale populations) and finally the social context (for example, the extent to which binge drinking is socially and politically acceptable). Imagine then the difficulties of measuring a concept such as patient safety.

The most commonly referred to definition of patient safety comes from the Institute of Medicine in the USA and is *freedom from accidental injury due to medical care or from medical error* (Institute of Medicine, 1999). The National Patient Safety Agency here in the UK had an alternative definition, describing patient safety as *the process by which an organisation makes patient care safer* (NPSA, 2004). But what does patient safety mean to healthcare staff and patients? When healthcare staff talk about safety, they may be referring to specific technical aspects of care such as drug allergies or catheter-related infections, whereas patients commonly raise issues of personal neglect, communication with staff and dignity as important priorities (Ward and Armitage, 2012). Thus, in the field of patient safety, a common definition and hence measurement tool may be more elusive.

What does a good measure look like?

Putting aside for one minute the complexity of measurement for patient safety, there are some common rules that help us decide what a good measure looks like. A good measure should:

- represent what it intends to measure (and is therefore valid);

- produce similar results when used repeatedly (is therefore reliable);

- be able to detect the phenomenon without being either over- or under-inclusive (have sensitivity and specificity);

- be affordable in economic cost and time;

- be usable for the person completing the measure and using the data.

We will look in more detail at each of these essential criteria for effective measurement. We will do this with reference to one particular measure of patient safety: the hospital standardised mortality ratio (HSMR). HSMR is an indicator of healthcare quality that measures whether the death rate at a hospital is higher or lower than you would expect. This is an improvement on a previous measure of organisational safety – crude death rates. Using crude death rates is neither a *valid* nor a *reliable* measure for many reasons, including the variation in death rates as a result of factors such as the size of the hospital, the local population, confounding single events (such as a flu epidemic), configuration of services (e.g. regional centre for intensive care, or regional centre for palliative care). What HSMRs have attempted to do is to take into account and adjust for at least some of these variations to provide a measure that allows comparison of death rates across organisations. However, a number of problems remain. Few statisticians believe it is possible for mortality ratios to capture the full complexity of variations in care, and doubt that the results are meaningful (Jarman *et al.*, 2010). This is all because of problems with validity (representing what it intends to measure), reliability (produces similar results when used repeatedly), sensitivity and specificity (detecting the phenomenon without being either over- or under-inclusive).

Validity

So, to establish whether HSMRs are good measures, the first question we need to ask is whether HSMRs are *valid* and measure what they intend to measure – patient safety at NHS trust level or at an organisational level. We would argue that the answer to this is no. Patients will inevitably die in hospital. In other words, although some of the harm is preventable, some is not and HSMRs do not distinguish (Pronovost and Colantuoni, 2009). Assuming that the definition of patient safety is the one provided by the Institute of Medicine, as described above, that is, *freedom from accidental injury due to medical care or from medical error* (Institute of Medicine, 2000, p4), HSMRs will also include deaths that are due not to medical care or error, but to unforeseeable and unpreventable events. Another indication that HSMRs may not be a valid measure of patient safety is that in some cases they have been found to be uncorrelated with alternative measures of patient safety. For example, in 2009, *Dr Foster's Hospital Guide* (**www.drfosterhealth.co.uk/docs/hospital-guide-2010. pdf**), based on HSMR, identified five hospitals as among the most improved over the past three years. Mid-Staffordshire NHS foundation trust was in the top five but at about the same time it was being branded by the Healthcare Commission (predecessor of the Care Quality Commission) as '*appalling*' (**www.cqc.org.uk/public/ reports-surveys-and-reviews/reports/cqc-annual-report-2010/11**).

Reliability

So, are HSMRs a *reliable* measure of patient safety, i.e. do they produce similar results when used repeatedly and across organisations? The answer again appears to be 'no'. This is a complex issue which we will not address in detail here; however, it is important to know that factors such as the way hospitals collect and code information about safety will differ between hospitals. Furthermore confounding factors such as service configuration and high rates of routine readmissions (revolving door patients) are not accounted for in the HSMR rates.

Sensitivity and specificity

Finally, we turn to the issue of sensitivity and specificity – that is, are HSMRs able to detect the phenomena (threats to safety) without being either over- or under-inclusive? Let us consider the common condition of asthma to help explain these terms. *Sensitivity* measures the proportion of correct cases identified as such (e.g. the percentage of people accurately diagnosed as having asthma). *Specificity* measures the proportion of non-cases which are correctly identified as such (e.g. the percentage of people without asthma who are correctly identified as not having the condition). However, there is always a trade-off in measurement between sensitivity and specificity. If you set the criteria too low you will diagnose most patients with breathing difficulties as having asthma (high sensitivity, low specificity). On the other hand, if a diagnosis of asthma was made only after a patient was admitted to accident and emergency with breathing difficulties that required oxygen, then you would be very likely to miss a large number of patients who have asthma (low sensitivity, high specificity). Although resources may be wasted when specificity is low, safety is enhanced by high sensitivity. Take the example of managing airline safety. It is essential to monitor continually for potential threats to safety. To this end, airport scanners may be set to alarm when encountering low-risk items like watches and coins (low specificity), to prevent the risk of overlooking items that pose a substantial threat to the aircraft and its passengers (high sensitivity).

In the context of measurement the same rules of sensitivity and specificity apply. The aviation industry does not use number of passengers lost inflight due to terrorism as a measure of airline safety (low sensitivity). Rather, it attempts to detect the number of threats to passenger safety during a flight which are far more common than aviation accidents, making the measure more sensitive. In the case of healthcare safety, deaths (the basis of HSMRs) represent only the tip of the iceberg while the mass of ice beneath the sea is represented by adverse events and near-misses.

The ratio of one major incident for every 300 minor incidents was first described by Herbert Heinrich in 1931 (Figure 7.1). Later work by Bird and Germain (1996) provided empirical support for this idea but suggested the ratio was more like 1 : 600. However, some have argued that this model assumes there is an inevitability that near-misses will eventually manifest as major incidents while others argue that a safe organisation can affect this ratio by putting in place defences (e.g. fail safe designs and processes) that absorb errors so they do not lead to harm (Conklin, 2007).

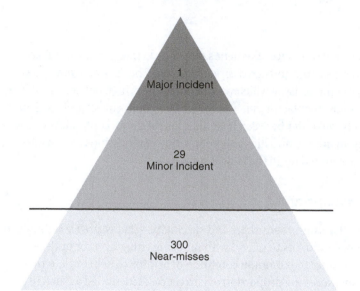

Figure 7.1 Heinrich's (1931) triangle, as it relates to patient safety.

If you really want to understand these arguments, see the 'Going further' section at the end of this chapter. Activity 7.2 will encourage you to reflect on the challenges of using HSMRs as a measurement of patient safety within your clinical practice.

ACTIVITY 7.2

During your next clinical placement, access the data about the HSMR for the trust in which you are working from Dr Foster's website (**www.drfosterhealth.co.uk/hospital-guide**) and reflect on the following.

1. Does your trust have a high or low HSMR compared to others in the region?
2. Think about your own experience and observations of the care and treatment processes in your placement and consider whether these might explain or alternatively be at odds with the published HSMR data.

So, now you have considered what HSMR data can tell us (or not) about patient safety and contrasted this with your own experience, the next step is to explore further measures of patient safety.

How do you measure patient safety?

In this section we will look at a variety of methods that are currently in use, including incident reporting, case note review and observation. We will then look at a different approach which involves measuring organisational structures and processes, and assessment of safety culture, rather than the adverse events themselves.

Incident reporting

Every trust must collect data on patient safety incidents (whether they be errors that result in near-misses, or adverse events) for the purposes of local and national monitoring, including both those events that are visible and (using the iceberg analogy) those that are below the surface. Incident reporting is often seen as the prime means of identifying the frequency and type of patient safety incidents, and of understanding the causes of these incidents. However, the quality of the data obtained from these reports depends on a number of factors, including the extent to which staff are willing and able to report events, the amount of information contained within the report (for example, about factors contributing to the incident) and the nature of the reporting scheme (for example, whether the reporting form is structured or unstructured, paper or electronic).

Activity 7.3 will help you to understand how the quality of information recorded in an incident report has an impact on the usefulness of these reports as a means of measuring and understanding patient safety incidents. It presents a verbatim incident report from a teaching hospital foundation trust in the UK.

You will note from Activity 7.3 that the quality of incident reporting is often poor. At the most basic level, there is still uncertainty amongst staff about what they should be reporting and many people only report events that have caused harm rather than any event that has the potential to cause harm and provide learning. To find out more about how to report, and the incidence and nature of patient safety incidents reported across the UK, you can access the National Reporting and Learning Scheme, set up by the National Patient Safety Agency (**www.nrls.npsa.nhs. uk/patient-safety-data/**). Of course, whether reporting is at a local or national level, many question the value of reporting as a measure of patient safety. Some of the problems with incident reporting are listed below.

ACTIVITY 7.3

I was about to give IV Tazocin as prescribed, when noticed that patient was allergic to penicillin. This was second dose, so one already given, await review. Cause: patient allergy. Action: copy to all involved and discussion with nurse concerned.

This is an actual report from an acute trust in which staff are asked to describe the incident, cause of the incident and the action taken to avoid further repetitions of the incident. Identify three ways in which it might be improved.

> ## What's the evidence?
>
> - You need to know what a patient safety incident is (and isn't) in order to report one (Allen and Barker, 1990). For example, if a staff nurse slips on a wet floor or is assaulted by a patient, this is not a patient safety incident.
> - Underreporting is the norm, particularly among doctors (Lawton and Parker, 2002; Armitage *et al.*, 2010), who may not perceive that reporting is part of their professional role.
> - The data in the report form are often scant and contain little risk-relevant information (Cantrill, 2006; National Patient Safety Agency, 2007).
> - Social desirability (the need to present oneself favourably) is a complication, meaning that people are reluctant to report events where they might be perceived to be incompetent.
> - Valuable incidents are in the eye of the beholder (Armitage and Chapman, 2007). So some may report any incident no matter whether harm has occurred, while others will only report incidents where there is observable patient harm.

Despite the problems, incident reporting does at least hold the potential for shared learning and remains a cost-effective way of collecting safety data compared with other methods, such as case note review and observation, which are discussed below.

Case note review

The Harvard Medical Practice Study (Brennan *et al.*, 1991) was the first large-scale investigation using case note review to identify medical errors. It was the starting point for a series of further studies which collectively provided compelling evidence for the existence of preventable harm (3.7 per cent of all hospital admissions result in preventable harm). Case notes are often a valuable source of detailed information about the process and outcomes of care and are routinely used by doctors to audit the safety of care. Using their professional judgment, clinicians may be able to identify and analyse patterns of care and errors. This approach is known as holistic or implicit case note review which relies on existing clinical knowledge and intuition. This contrasts with criterion-based or explicit case note review which allows comparison of care against explicit standards (for example, a national clinical guideline such as the optimum treatment for asthma, as detailed by the British Thoracic Society, 2012). This explicit method of case note review reduces the risk of subjectivity and any resulting bias. So, if two health professionals analyse case notes using this second explicit approach, they are much more likely to agree on the existence of adverse events and errors. This level of agreement between the two health professionals is referred to as interrater reliability. Like incident reporting, case note review also has a number of limitations, which include:

- the time-consuming and costly nature of data collection (Hutchinson *et al.*, 2010 found that it takes trained clinicians a mean average of 18 minutes to conduct a holistic review, costing over £10 for a doctor per review);

- case note review is vulnerable to an individual's particular perception of the existence of preventable harm (Runciman *et al.*, 2003); clinicians may not agree that a decubitus ulcer is always the result of a failure in care but can be an inevitable complication in an elderly, immobile patient with multiple comorbidities;

- identifying near-misses is often difficult due to the incompleteness of the case notes (Wald and Shojania, 2003; Adisasmita *et al.*, 2008).

Junior doctors may find themselves invited to a routine case note review meeting when a clinical unit assesses compliance with National Institute for Health and Clinical Excellence standards or another notable benchmark of quality.

Observation

Observation is the other principal research method in the detection of error and adverse events (and so measurement of patient safety). One of the most cited observational studies is that of Andrews *et al.* (1997), who used trained qualitative observers in a study of adverse events in a North American general hospital. They attended day shifts, handovers, notable departmental meetings and case conferences, concluding that 185 out of 1,047 (17.7 per cent) patients had suffered at least one serious adverse event. Critically, the adverse event incidence proved to be much higher than in studies employing non-observational methods such as case note review (see above). As well as identifying the incidence of preventable harm, observation can be used to identify the causes of harm. In a study of intravenous medication errors (Taxis and Barber, 2003), a very structured observation process led to a calculation of the type and clinical importance of the errors. The observers accompanied nurses in their drug administration activities, but the nurses were not told of the true purpose of the study so as to reduce the Hawthorne effect (the impact of the researcher on the observed participant's behaviour). Whilst reducing the Hawthorne effect is useful for the collection of valid data, it also arguably threatens the autonomy of the observed participants, an ethical consideration which has been explored elsewhere (Armitage, 2005). Although Lilford *et al.* (2003) have described observation as the gold standard in the detection of preventable harm, this method does have a number of challenges.

- Observation is an expensive method because one or more people with clinical expertise must watch and carefully document clinical practice over a long period of time.

- Well-trained observers are required to ensure reliability and consistency.

- For these reasons, observation is not feasible for capturing rarely occurring events (Thomas and Petersen, 2003).

Measurement of structures and processes

Eminent patient safety researchers (such as Charles Vincent, 2010) have concluded that there is no perfect way of estimating the incidence of adverse events or errors. With this in mind, some authors (Battles and Lilford, 2003; Pronovost *et al.*, 2006) have argued against a focus solely on adverse events or other outcomes and instead point to the role of organisational structures and processes of care in contributing to patient safety incidents. This argument for a focus on the measurement of structures and processes as well as outcomes is not new and in fact was first proposed by Donabedian (1980) in relation to the monitoring of quality (Figure 7.2).

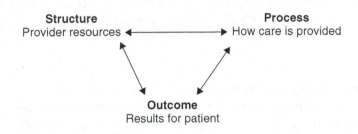

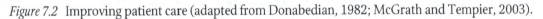

Figure 7.2 Improving patient care (adapted from Donabedian, 1982; McGrath and Tempier, 2003).

Historically, clinicians have argued that risk and harm are inevitable. This view has changed and it may even be argued that all harm is preventable (Pronovost and Colantuoni, 2009). However, this distinction between preventable and inevitable harm is often unclear as it is susceptible to individual judgment and advances in practice. Thus, many have turned to the measurement of a process as an alternative way of measuring patient safety. The fundamental advantage of measuring process (how care is provided at individual or organisational levels) rather than outcome is an acknowledgment of the inevitable variation in the patient's condition. For example, numbers of cardiac arrests will vary as a function of the patient's condition and location, being more likely among an elderly population in a critical care unit, which means that recording the differing numbers of cardiac arrests across hospital units is unlikely to be a valid measure of patient safety. On the other hand, measuring the proportion of patients with a modified early warning score (MEWS) of 5 who are assessed by a critical care team (a process measure) allows comparison across patient populations and locations. However, to be a valid measure of process there must be strong evidence of a direct causal (rather than assumed) relationship to a specific outcome. In a review published in the *Journal of the American Medical Association*, Leape *et al.* (2002) identified those processes (referred to as patient safety practices) where there is strong evidence that compliance with these safety practices significantly reduces the risk of preventable harm and where the risks of implementing them are low. These are listed in the following 'What's the evidence?' box.

What's the evidence?

Table 7.1 Patient safety practices

Strongest level of evidence that they lead to better patient outcomes	Weak level of evidence but potentially high-impact practices
Ultrasound-guided central venous line insertion Automatic stop orders with urinary catheters (remove after 48–72 hours) Prevention of catheter-related bloodstream infection through specific sterile procedures (hand hygiene; maximum sterile barrier; chlorhexidine rather than iodine for skin preparation; avoiding femoral site; prompt removal) Read back for high-priority communications and laboratory results	Post-discharge telephone follow-up telephone calls Structured handover communications Structured discharge summaries (complete medication list; any new diagnosis; pending investigations)

(Source: adapted from Leape *et al.*, 2002 and Ranji and Shojaniah, 2008.)

Finally, there are variations in structure. These exist at the *whole* organisational level and are embedded within healthcare systems, which, although less visible and proximal to patient safety outcomes, inevitably contribute to harm. These include factors such as the procurement and supply of equipment, the design of care pathways and the nature of clinical handovers. One of the advantages of measuring structural variables is that it acknowledges the vulnerability of health professionals working at the sharp end of practice to error when the conditions do not support safe practice. Quoting from Reason (1997), *we cannot change the human condition but we can change the conditions in which people work.*

ACTIVITY 7.4

You are working on a ward where the majority of patients are elderly, immobile and have a poor nutritional status and problems with continence. You recognise that these patients are vulnerable to pressure ulcers but that some patients are admitted with pre-existing ulcers.

1. Will focusing simply on outcome measures (number of patients with pressure ulcers) provide a valid measure of patient safety here?

2. What process measures could be considered?

3. What structure measures might you also want to record?

Answers

1. No, because some wards might have more patients who are admitted with pre-existing ulcers.

2. Recording of pressure ulcer severity (using a published scale) and treatment plans in the patient notes.

3. Whether or not pressure-relieving mattresses are available for patients.

Assessment of safety culture/measuring safety culture

A quite different approach to the measurement of patient safety in healthcare organisations that has grown in popularity over the last ten years is the assessment of safety culture. However, little agreement exists about whether or not safety culture can be measured, depending on the definition of the term. Safety culture is commonly referred to as a set of shared values and beliefs or *the way we do things around here* (Schein, 1992, p9). This might be illustrated by a maternity unit routinely reviewing the case notes for each delivery each week, in a rotating multidisciplinary team, as a mandatory part of practice. Scott *et al.* (2003) explain that measurement should focus on specific variables (such as incident-reporting processes) or upon intrinsic properties of the social environment (such as conflict or co-operation). However, these manifestations of group values are difficult constructs to measure, so many have opted for the quantitative measurement of safety attitudes (as in measures of safety climate: Flin *et al.*, 2000) as an alternative.

Regulatory bodies such as the Joint Commission in the USA and the Health and Safety Executive have readily adopted such measures but there is little evidence of their precision and accuracy, specifically their reliability and validity, as discussed earlier in this chapter (Flin, 2007). To address these concerns it is now recommended that quantitative data are supplemented by contextual qualitative data (through, for example, observations and interviews) to gain a fuller understanding (Halligan and Zecevic, 2011). An alternative approach is to assess cultural maturity (whether a group manages safety as an integral part of all its activities and patient involvement is well established), through a whole-team approach, and ultimately to develop an improvement strategy (**www.nrls.npsa.nhs.uk/resources/?entryid45=59796**). It is worth bearing in mind, however, that there is little evidence that a strong culture, whatever the measure, leads to a strong performance (Scott *et al.*, 2003).

How can measurement help in my practice?

Measurement serves many goals: describing the status quo, measuring improvement and motivating change. The kind of measurement tools and methods that are utilised depends on the purpose. For example, a research study might necessitate the systematic collection of large amounts of data from across a wide range of patient populations to calculate a significant difference between groups (e.g. experimental and control). On the other hand, a quality improvement project may simply require the recording of an activity on a limited number of occasions to demonstrate a trend or pattern. Thus, the way data is collected, analysed and applied is dependent on the goal of the measurement.

Measurement is a strong motivator for individual change. Imagine that you want to reduce your chance of heart disease (outcome). There is good evidence that being more physically active (process) can help to reduce your risk of heart disease, and that walking 20,000 steps a day represents a good level of physical activity. Evidence suggests that one of the best ways of encouraging people to be more active is to ask them to monitor their activity on a daily basis, in other words to measure their performance continuously. This monitoring (and feedback) can be used to promote changes in performance/behaviour that serve a variety of goals, including safety.

That improvement cannot happen without measurement is the underlying philosophy of many team-based quality and safety improvement activities. In a training programme known as Training and Action for Patient Safety (TAPS), recently developed as part of the Yorkshire and Humber Health Innovation and Education Cluster, this is the guiding principle. Multiprofessional teams come together to address a patient safety problem in their unit. However, in order to demonstrate both that the problem exists and that the solution (often a structural or process change) has been effective, the teams must continuously measure both processes and outcomes. The case study gives an example of this in action at a GP training practice in Sheffield.

Case Study: TAPS for improving the assessment of sick children at a GP Training Practice in Sheffield

Aim

The aim was to improve the assessment of sick children by ensuring: (1) that all children under three years old presenting with an acute illness are assessed and managed according to the National Institute for Health and Clinical Excellence (NICE) guidelines for feverish illness in children; and (2) that clinicians are providing care appropriate to their level of competence.

Problem

Sick children may be seen by a GP, GP trainee or prescribing nurse (backup systems exist for a second opinion from an experienced GP), but GP registrars may not have had experience of working in paediatrics and nurses were concerned about whether they are appropriately trained for this.

Actions

After reviewing the problem the multiprofessional team identified actions to improve assessment of sick children within the practice. This included creation of an assessment template based on NICE guidelines and a traffic light system within the practice computer system. Training was provided for all clinical staff, including face-to-face meetings with anyone not present at the initial meeting. Locum staff were also inducted into the new system and discussions held with anyone not using the template.

Results

Initially 14 per cent of clinicians were conforming to NICE guidance but by the end of the programme 90 per cent were recording all four NICE guideline parameters in a patient's record and 100 per cent had documented an appropriate safety net.

Learning and impact

The TAPS programme has enabled the practice to implement a safer system for assessing sick children according to NICE guidelines. To ensure sustainability, the practice plans to audit the system periodically to ensure it is still effective.

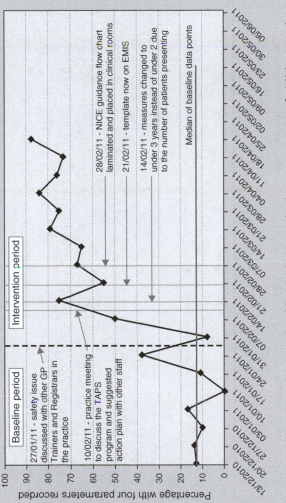

Figure 7.3 Medical Centre, Sheffield. Measure 1: the percentage of children under three presenting with an acute illness who have had recorded the four parameters recommended by NICE.

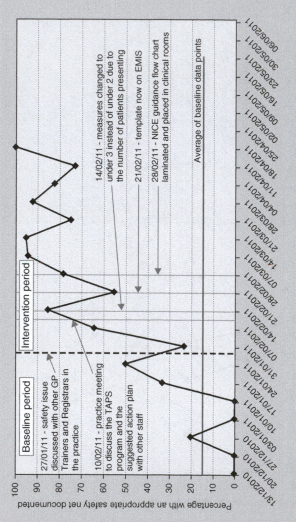

Figure 7.4 Medical Centre, Sheffield. Measure 2: the percentage of children under three presenting with an acute illness who have had an appropriate safety net documented in their records.

Measurement is also a means of throwing into stark relief a problem that is recognised at a local level but that requires recognition at an organisational level and also support for a solution. Thus, measurement serves as a driver for organisational accountability for safety. Although there are currently few measurement tools available, work is now underway within the Quality and Safety Research group at the Bradford Institute for Health Research to develop a tool that will facilitate the measurement of safety at an organisational level.

You may therefore be involved in the measurement of patient safety in several ways. You might carry out measurement alone or as part of a peer group for a specific educational programme, or perhaps as a foundation doctor in a multidisciplinary team. You may need to select an appropriate measure (or range of measures) for a particular purpose, and be able to comment on strengths and weaknesses, reliability and cost.

ACTIVITY 7.5

Read and reflect upon the case study below. Imagine that you were the junior doctor and consider:

1. What where the threats to patient safety?
2. At least two possible strategies that might reduce these threats.
3. At least one measure (for each strategy) that would help you to identify whether your strategy had worked.
4. Whether each of your measures is a structure, process or outcome measure.

Case Study

A patient has been transferred to the High Dependency Unit with pneumonia. The patient had deteriorating observations for four hours on the ward before a senior medical review and appropriate transfer occurred. There is an early-warning policy in place at this hospital. The patient was under the care of the general medical consultant. Unfortunately no bed was available in the appropriate specialty so the medical patient was 'lodged' on a urology ward due to an episode of vomiting and thought to need isolation in a side room. The nurse had recorded the patient's routine observations and alerted the ward junior doctor to the patient's low oxygen saturations (while on oxygen therapy), temperature and increasing heart rate.

The new junior doctor was not aware of the early-warning policy covering patient deterioration and the ward was using a traditional observation chart rather than one which incorporated the recording of a medical early warning system (MEWS) protocol. The junior doctor assessed the patient and arranged basic investigations.

Despite the patient having developed low blood pressure, the junior doctor did not escalate to a senior member of staff for a further 60 minutes. The junior doctor had spent time trying to identify which consultant the patient was under before being able to contact the appropriate registrar to review. Consequently the patient's deterioration was detected but not acted upon.

The case study you have been looking at was based on a real adverse event in a hospital trust. The patient's condition was not unusual but, as is often the case, the care given was poor as a result of several systems failures. Healthcare organisations are frequently required to undertake detailed investigations of such incidents in an attempt to identify their contributory factors and reduce the likelihood of similar events occurring. You have identified the contributory factors in this case but additionally considered how the patient's care could have been improved, and how any improvement could be demonstrated through effective measurement.

Chapter summary

If we want to know how well we are doing (whether as a healthcare system, organisation or team) in patient safety then effective measurement is necessary. In this chapter we argue that there is no definitive measure of patient safety, but that appropriate measurement depends on the *definition of patient safety* and the *purpose of the measurement*. Despite there being no single way of measuring safety there are specific questions one should ask when choosing a measure: does it measure what I want it to measure, is it sufficiently sensitive and will it provide reliable data? In other words, does your measurement tool measure precisely what you intend to measure and, if used repeatedly, will it provide similar results?

Common measures of patient safety tend to identify instances when things have gone wrong, for example through incident reporting, case note review or observation. So they focus on negative outcomes. Here we argue that the measurement of outcomes in the form of incidents and near-misses is fraught with problems and that measurement of process should be encouraged, especially where there is strong evidence that a particular process affects an outcome. We also introduce other forms of patient safety measurement that focus on a subjective understanding of patient safety values, beliefs and behaviour among staff – a culture of safety.

The measurement of patient safety is challenging but when carefully planned and implemented, measurement remains a strong stimulus for change, and is essential for demonstrating both failure and improvement.

GOING FURTHER

Vincent, C (2010) *Patient Safety*, 2nd edition. London: Wiley Blackwell/BMJ Books. Charles Vincent has written an excellent and very readable section on measurement in the latest edition of this book. Professor Vincent addresses some of the topics covered in this chapter, but from a different perspective, which should serve to increase your understanding of measurement.

There are several pocket books on quality improvement methods which can provide useful information on easily implemented measures, many of which are applicable to patient safety improvements. The *1000 Lives O Fywydau Quality Improvement Guide* from NHS Wales is an excellent example. The guide differentiates between the different data requirements when measuring for research, accountability or quality improvement, and provides helpful information on planning for what is to be accomplished, how any change in practice might be demonstrated to be an improvement, and how change can be introduced. It is available at: **www.wales.nhs.uk/sites3/page.cfm?orgid=781&pid=52913**.

If you would like more information about HSMRs and their analysis, go to: **www.straightstatistics.org/article/coding-maze-mortality-ratios-and-real-life**.

Measuring mortality is also covered by Professor Sir Brian Jarman and others in the Dr Foster *Test Results*. This easy-to-follow online publication additionally offers a section on patient safety (Chapter 26) which describes some of the inconsistencies in defining, recording and measuring frequency of venous thromboembolisms. See **www.drfosterhealth.co.uk/docs/hospital-guide-2010.pdf**.

References

Aasland, OG and Forde, R (2005) Impact of feeling responsible for adverse events on doctors' personal and professional lives: the importance of being open to criticism from colleagues. *Quality and Safety in Healthcare,* 14: 13–17.

Action against Medical Accidents (2011) *Response to Listening Exercise on Health and Social Care Bill.* www.avma.org.uk/data/files/avmarelisteningexercise.pdf.

Adisasmita, A, Deviany, PE, Nandiaty, F, Stanton, C and Ronsmans, C (2008) Obstetric near miss and deaths in public and private hospitals in Indonesia. *BMC Pregnancy and Childbirth,* 8(1): 1.

Alimo-Metcalf, B and Alban-Metcalf, J (2002) Leadership, in Warr, P (ed.) *Psychology at Work.* London: Penguin, pp. 300–25.

Allen, EL and Barker, KN (1990) Fundamentals of medication error research. *American Journal of Hospital Pharmacy,* 47: 555–71.

Amabile, TM and Khaire, M (2008) Creativity and the role of the leader. *Harvard Business Review,* Reprint order R0810G. Accessed at www.hbr.org. on 31 October 2011.

Anderson, N and West, M (1998) Measuring climate for work group innovation: development and validation of the team climate inventory. *Journal of Organisational Behavior,* 19: 235–58.

Andrews, LB, Stocking, C, Krizek, T, Gottlieb, L, Krizek, C, Vargish, T and Siegler, M (1997) An alternative strategy for studying adverse events in medical care. *Lancet,* 349(9048): 309–13.

Armitage, G (2005) Drug errors, qualitative research and some reflections on ethics. *Journal of Clinical Nursing,* 14: 869–75.

Armitage, G and Chapman, EJ (2007) Incident reporting: a curate's egg? *Journal of Integrated Care Pathways,* 10: 92–6.

Armitage, G, Newell, RJ and Wright, J (2010) Improving drug error reporting. *Journal of Evaluation in Clinical Practice,* 16(I6): 118–19.

Attree, M (2007) Factors influencing nurses' decisions to raise concerns about care quality. *Journal of Nursing Management,* 15: 392–402.

Bangor, A, Kortum, PT and Miller, JT (2008) An empirical evaluation of the system usability scale. *International Journal of Human–Computer Interaction,* 24: 574–94.

Barez-Brown, C (2011) *Shine: How to survive and thrive at work.* London: Penguin.

Bate, P and Robert, G (2006) Experience-based design: from designing the system around the patient to co-designing services with the patient. *Quality and Safety in Health Care*, 15(5): 307–10.

Battles, J and Lilford, R (2003) Organizing patient safety research to identify risks and hazards. *BMJ Quality and Safety in Health Care*, 12: ii2–7.

Berridge, V, Herring, R and Thom, B (2009) Binge drinking: a confused concept and its contemporary history. *Social History of Medicine*, 22(3): 597–607.

Besco, RO (1999) PACE: probe, alert, challenge, and emergency action. *Business and Commercial Aviation*, 84(6): 72–4.

Bird, F and Germain, G (1996) *Loss Control Management: Practical loss control leadership*, revised edition. Loganville: Det Norske Veritas (USA).

Birkinshaw, J, Bouquet, C and Barsoux, J (2011) The 5 myths of innovation. *MIT Sloan Management Review*, Winter: 1–8.

Blenkinsopp, A, Wilkie, P, Wang, M and Routledge, PA (2006) Patient reporting of suspected adverse drug reactions: a review of published literature and international experience. *British Journal of Clinical Pharmacology*, 63: 148–56.

Botwinick, L, Bisogagno, M and Haraden, C (2006) *Leadership Guide to Patient Safety*, IHI Innovation Series. Cambridge, MA: Institute for Healthcare Improvement.

Brennan, TA, Leape, LL, Laird, NM, Lawthers, AG, Localio, AR, Barnes, BA, Hebert, L *et al.* (1991) Incidence of adverse events and negligence in hospitalized patients: results of the Harvard Medical Practice Study I. *New England Journal of Medicine*, 324: 370–6.

British Thoracic Society (2012) British Guideline on the Management of Asthma.www.brit-thoracic.org.uk/Portals/0/Guidelines/AsthmaGuidelines/sign101%20Jan%202012.pdf.

Brooke, J (1996) SUS: A 'quick and dirty' usability scale, in Jordan, PW, Thomas, B, Weerdmeester, BA and McClelland, IL (eds) *Usability Evaluation in Industry*. London: Taylor and Francis.

Cantrill, J (2006) *Medication Error 2. Patient Safety Research Portfolio: Development of capacity and evaluation of IT solutions.* Birmingham: Department of Public Health and Epidemiology, Birmingham University.

Carayon, P, Schoofs Hundt, A, Karsh, B-T, Gurses, AP, Alvarado, CJ, Smith, M and Flatley Brennan, P (2006) Work system design for patient safety: the SEIPS model. *Quality and Safety in Health Care*, 15 (suppl. I): i50–8.

Carthey, J and Clarke, J (2009) The 'how to guide' for implementing human factors in healthcare. *Patient Safety First*. www.patientsafetyfirst.nhs.uk.

Catwell, L and Sheikh, A (2009) Evaluating eHealth interventions: the need for continuous systemic evaluation. *PLoS Medicine*, 6(8): e1000126.

Chan, J, Shojania, KG, Easty, AC and Etchells, EE (2011) Usability evaluation of order sets in a computerised provider order entry system. *BMJ Quality and Safety*, 20: 932–40.

Chiarella, M and McInnes, E (2008) Legality, morality and reality – the role of the nurse in maintaining standards of care. *Australian Journal of Advanced Nursing*, 26(1): 77–109.

Christensen, CM, Dyer, J and Gregerson, H (2011) *The Innovator's DNA: Mastering the five skills of disruptive innovators.* Boston, MA: Harvard Business School Press.

Classen, DC, Lloyd, RC, Provost, L, Griffin, FA and Resar, R (2008) Development and evaluation of the Institute for Healthcare Improvement Global Trigger Tool. *Journal of Patient Safety*, 4(3): 169–77.

Cohen, ER, Feinglass, J, Barsuk, JH, Barnard, C, O'Donnell, A, McGaghie, WC and Wayne, DB (2010) Cost savings from reduced catheter-related bloodstream infection after simulation-based education for residents in a medical intensive care unit. *Simulated Healthcare*, 5(2): 98–102.

Conklin, T (2007) Preventing serious accidents with the human performance philosophy. *Nuclear Weapons Journal*, 1: 17–18.

Cooper-Patrick, L, Gallo, JJ, Gonzales, JJ, Thi Vu, H, Powe, NR, Nelson, C, Ford, DE *et al.* (1999) Race, gender and partnership in the patient–physician relationship. *Journal of the American Medical Assocation*, 282: 583–9.

Cousins, D (2007) *Safety in Doses: Improving the Use of Medicines in the NHS.* London: National Patient Safety Agency.

Croskerry, P (2009a) A universal model of diagnostic reasoning. *Academic Medicine*, 84: 1022–8.

Croskerry, P (2009b) Clinical cognition and diagnostic error: applications of a dual process model of reasoning. *Advances in Health Sciences Education*, 14: 27–35.

Curtis, K, Tzannes, A and Rudge, T (2011) How to talk to doctors – a guide for effective communication. *International Nursing Review*, 58: 13–20.

Davis, RE, Koutantji, M and Vincent, CA (2008) How willing are patients to question healthcare staff on issues related to the quality and safety of their healthcare? An exploratory study. *Quality and Safety in Health Care*, 17: 90–6.

Davis, RE, Sevdalis, N and Vincent, CA (2011) Patient involvement in patient safety: how willing are patients to participate? *BMJ Quality and Safety*, 20: 108–14.

deBono, E (1990) *Lateral Thinking.* London: Penguin.

deBono, E (2007) *How to Have Creative Ideas.* London: Vermilion.

deBono, E (2010) *Thinking Course, Powerful Tools to Transform your Thinking.* Harlow: BBC.

Department of Health (1998) *A First Class Service: Quality in the new NHS.* London: HMSO.

Department of Health (2000) *An Organisation with a Memory.* London: The Stationery Office.

Department of Health (2004) *Patient and Public Involvement in Health: The evidence for policy implementation.* London: The Stationery Office.

Department of Health (2005) *Creating a Patient-led NHS: Delivering the NHS improvement plan.* London: Department of Health.

Department of Health (2008) *High Quality Care for All: NHS next stage review* (the Darzi Report). London: Department of Health.

Department of Health (2010a) *Equity and Excellence: Liberating the NHS.* London: The Stationery Office.

Department of Health (2010b) *The NHS Constitution for England.* London: The Stationery Office.

Department of Health (2011a) *Quality, Innovation, Production, Prevention (QIPP) programme.* www.institute.nhs.uk/cost_and_quality/qipp/cost_and_quality_homepage.html.

Department of Health (2011b) *The Foundation Programme Curriculum.* London: Office of Public Sector Information.

De Vries, EN, Ramrattan, MA, Smorenburg, SM, Gouma, DJ and Boermeester, MA (2008) The incidence and nature of in-hospital adverse events: a systematic review. *Quality and Safety in Health Care,* 17: 216–23.

Divi, C, Koss, RG, Schmaltz, SP and Loeb, JM (2007) Language proficiency and adverse events in U.S. hospitals: a pilot study. *International Journal of Quality Health Care,* 19: 60–7.

Donabedian, A (1980) *The Definition of Quality and Approaches to its Assessment.* Ann Arbor, MI: Health Administration Press.

Donabedian, A (1992) The Lichfield lecture. Quality assurance in health care: the consumer's role. *Quality in Health Care,* 1(4): 247–51.

Donaldson, LJ (2008) Put the patient in the room, always. *Quality and Safety in Health Care,* 17: 82–3.

Dornan, T, Ashcroft, D, Heathfield, H, Lewis, P, Miles, J, Taylor, D, Tully, M and Wass, V (2009) *An In depth Investigation into Causes of Prescribing Errors by Foundation Trainees in Relation to their Medical Education: EQUIP study.* London: General Medical Council.

Egberts, TCG, Smulders, M, de Koning, FHP, Meyboom, RHB and Leufkens, HGM (1996) Can adverse drug reactions be detected earlier? A comparison of reports by patients and professionals. *British Medical Journal,* 313: 530–1.

Entwistle, V (2007) Differing perspectives on patient involvement in patient safety. *Quality and Safety in Health Care*, 16: 140–2.

Entwistle, VA, Mello, MM and Brennan, TA (2005) Advising patients about patient safety: current initiatives risk shifting responsibility. *Joint Commission Journal on Quality and Safety in Health Care*, 31: 483–94.

Entwistle, VA, McCaughan, D, Watt, I, Birks, Y, Hall, J, Peat, M, Williams, B *et al.* (2010) Speaking up about safety concerns: multi-setting qualitative study of patients' views and experiences. *Quality and Safety in Health Care*, 19: e33.

Fagin, L and Garelick, A (2004) The doctor–nurse relationship. *Psychiatric Treatment*, 10: 277–86.

Fairbanks, RJ, Caplan, SH, Bishop, PA, Marks, AM and Shah, MN (2007) Usability study of two common defibrillators reveals hazards. *Annals of Emergency Medicine*, 50(4): 424–32.

Firth-Cozens, J (2001a) Multidisciplinary teamwork: the good, bad, and everything in between. *Quality in Health Care*, 10(2): 65.

Firth-Cozens, J (2001b) Cultures for improving patient safety through learning: the role of teamwork. *Quality in Health Care*, 10 (suppl. II): ii26–31.

Fisseni, G, Pentzek, M and Abholz, H (2007) Responding to serious medical error in general practice consequences for the GPs involved: analysis of 75 cases from Germany. *Family Practice*, 71: 9–13.

Flin, R (2007) Measuring safety culture in healthcare: a case for accurate diagnosis. *Safety Science*, 45: 653–67.

Flin, R and Patey, R (2009) Training in non-technical skills to improve patient safety. *British Medical Journal*, 339: 985–6.

Flin, R, Mearns, K, O'Conner, P and Bryden, R (2000) Measuring safety climate: identifying the common features. *Safety Science*, 34: 177–92.

Franklin, DB, Birch, S, Savage, I, Wong, I, Woloshynowych, M, Jacklin, A and Barber, N (2009) Methodological variability in detecting prescribing errors and consequences for the evaluation of interventions. *Pharmacoepidemiology and Drug Safety*, 18: 981–1123.

Frey, B, Ersch, J, Bernet, V, Baenziger, O, Enderli, L and Doell, C (2009) Involvement of parents in critical incidents in a neo-natal-paediatric intensive care unit. *Quality and Safety in Health Care*, 18: 446–9.

Gallagher, TH, Waterman, AD, Ebers, AG, Fraser, VJ and Levinson, W (2003) Patients' physicians' attitudes regarding the disclosure of medical errors. *Journal of the American Medical Association*, 289: 1001–7.

Garrett, PW, Dickson, HG, Young, L and Whelan, AK (2008) 'The happy migrant effect': perceptions of negative experiences of healthcare by patients with little or no English: a qualitative study across seven language groups. *Quality and Safety in Health Care,* 17: 101–3.

General Medical Council (2009a) *Tomorrow's Doctors.* www.gmc-uk.org/ education/undergraduate/tomorrows_doctors_2009.asp.

General Medical Council (2009b) *Good Medical Practice.*

General Medical Council (2011) *The Trainee Doctor: Foundation and specialty, including GP training.* London: GMC.

Gerrish, K and Papadopolous, I (1999) Transcultural competence: the challenge for nurse education. *British Journal of Nursing,* 8: 1453–7.

Granville, G (2006) *What Does the Service Improvement Literature Tell Us and How Can It Make a Difference to Implementation?* Accessed at www.gilliangranville. com on 31 October 2011.

Greenfield, D, Nugus, P, Travaglia, J and Braithwaite, J (2011) Factors that shape the development of interprofessional improvement initiatives in health organisations. *BMJ Quality and Safety,* 20(4): 332–7.

Gawande, A (2011) *The Checklist Manifesto: How to get things right.* London: Profile Books.

Halligan, M and Zecevic, A (2011) Safety culture in healthcare: a review of concepts, dimensions, measures and progress. *BMJ Quality and Safety in Healthcare,* 20: 338–43.

Haynes, AB, Weiser, TG, Berry, WR, Lipsitz, SR, Breizat, AS, Patchen Dellinger, E, Herbosa, T *et al.* (2009) A surgical checklist to reduce morbidity and mortality in a global population. *New England Journal of Medicine,* 360: 491–9.

Haynes, AB, Weiser, TG, Berry, WR, Lipsitz, SR, Breizat, AS, Patchen Dellinger, E, Dzeiken, G *et al.* (2011). Changes in safety attitude and relationship to decreased postoperative morbidity and mortality following implementation of a checklist-based surgical safety intervention. *BMJ Quality and Safety,* 20: 102–7.

Health Foundation (2011) *Evaluating Healthcare Quality Improvement.* Accessed at www.health.org.uk/publications/evaluating-healthcare-quality-improvement/ on 25 May 2012.

Heinrich, HW (1931). *Industrial Accident Prevention: A scientific approach.* New York: McGraw-Hill.

Helmreich, RL (2000) On error management: lessons from aviation. *British Medical Journal,* 320 (7237): 781–5.

Henderson, S (2003) Power imbalance between nurses and patients: a potential inhibitor of partnership in care. *Journal of Clinical Nursing,* 12: 501–8.

Heritage, J, Robinson, JD, Elliott, MN, Beckett, M and Wilkes, M (2006) Reducing patients' unmet concerns in primary care: the difference one word can make. *Journal of General Internal Medicine,* 22(10): 1429–33.

Hibbard, JH, Peters, E, Slovic, P and Tusler, M (2005) Can patients be part of the solution? Views on their role in preventing medical errors. *Medical Care Research and Review*, 62: 601–16.

House of Commons Health Committee (2009) *Patient Safety: Sixth Report of Session 2008–09.* London: The Stationery Office.

Hunt, EA, Shilkofski, NA, Stavroudis, TA and Nelson, KL *(2007)* Simulation: translation to improved team performance. *Anesthesiology Clinics*, 25(2): 301–19.

Hutchinson, A, Coster, JE, Cooper, KL, McIntosh, A, Walters, SJ, Bath, PA, Pearson, M *et al*. (2010) Comparison of case note review methods for evaluating quality and safety in health care. *NIHR / Health Technology Assessment Programme*, February DOI: 10.3310/hta14100.

Institute of Medicine (1999) *To Err is Human: Building a safer health system.* Washington, DC: National Academy Press.

International Alliance of Patient Organisations (2005) *Policy Statement: Patient Involvement.* www.patientsorganizations.org, accessed 9 October 2011.

International Ergonomics Association (2000) *What is Ergonomics?* www.iea.cc/.

International Organization for Standardization (1998). *ISO 9241–11 Ergonomic Requirements for Office Work with Visual Display Terminals (VDTs) – Part II: Guidance on usability*. Geneva: International Organization for Standardization.

Jacobson, B and Murray, A (2007) *Medical Devices: Use and safety*. Edinburgh: Churchill Livingstone.

Jarman, B, Aylin, P and Bottle, A (2010) Hospital mortality ratios. A plea for reason. *British Medical Journal*, 340: c2744.

Jha, V, Quinton, ND, Bekker, HL and Roberts, TE (2009) Strategies and interventions for involvement of real patients in medical education: a systematic review. *Medical Education*, 43: 10–20.

Jirwe, M, Gerrish, K, Keeney, S and Emami, A (2009) Identifying the core components of cultural competence: findings from a Delphi study. *Journal of Clinical Nursing*, 18: 2622–34.

Johnstone, MJ and Kanistaki, O (2009) Engaging patients as safety partners: some considerations for ensuring a culturally and linguistically appropriate approach. *Health Policy*, 90: 1–7.

Joosten, EAG, DeFuentes-Merillas, L, de Weert, GH, Sensky, T, van der Staak, CPF and de Jong, CAJ (2008) Systematic review of the effects of shared decision-making on patient satisfaction, treatment adherence and health status. *Psychotherapy and Psychosomatics*, 77: 219–26.

Kaboli, PJ, Glasgow, JM, Komal Jaipul, C, Barry, WA, Strayer, JR, Mutnick, B and Rosenthal, GE (2010) Identifying medication misadventures: poor agreement among medical record, physician, nurse and patient reports. *Pharmacotherapy*, 30: 529–38.

Kelley, T and Littleman, J (2004) *The Art of Innovation.* London: Profile Books.

Kennedy, R, Lawless, M and Slater, B (2009) The ten essentials of large-scale change. *British Journal of Healthcare Management*, 15(11): 484–8.

King, A, Daniels, J, Lim, J, Cochrane, DD, Taylor, A and Ansermino, JM (2010) Time to listen: a review of methods to solicit patient reports of adverse events. *Quality and Safety in Health Care*, 19: 148–57.

Koppel, R, Metlay, JP, Cohen, A, Abaluck, B, Localio, AR, Kimmel, SE and Strom, BL (2005) Role of computerized physician order entry systems in facilitating medication errors. *Journal of the American Medical Association*, 293(10): 1197–203.

Koutantji, M, Davis, R, Vincent, CA and Coulter, A (2005) The patient's role in patient safety: engaging patients, their representatives, and health professionals. *Clinical Risk*, 11: 99–104.

Krause, SS (2003) *Aircraft Safety: Accident investigations, analyses and applications*, 2nd edition. New York: McGraw Hill.

Langley, G, Nolan, K, Nolan, T, Norman, C and Provost, L (2009) *The Improvement Guide: A practical approach to enhancing organisational performance*, 2nd edition. San Francisco: Jossey-Bass.

Lansley, A (2011) www.healthcareinnovationexpo.com/images/library/files/ 2010%20keynote%20speech/lansleyspeech.doc, accessed 9 October 2011.

Lawton, R and Parker, D (2002) Barriers to incident reporting in a healthcare system. *Quality and Safety in Health Care*, 11: 15–18.

Lawton, RJ, Gardner, PH, Green, BJ, Davey, C, Chamberlain, P, Phillips, P and Hughes, G (2009) An engineered solution to the maladministration of spinal injections. *Quality and Safety in Health Care*, 18: 492–5.

Leape, L, Berwick, DM and Bates, DW (2002) What practices will most improve safety? Evidence-based medicine meets patient safety. *Journal of the American Medical Association*, 288(4): 501–7.

Leape, L, Berwick, D, Clancy, C, Conway, J, Gluck, P, Guest, J, Lawrence, D *et al.* (2009) Transforming healthcare: a safety imperative. *Quality and Safety in Health Care*, 18: 424–8.

Leistikow, I, Kalkman, CJ, and Bruijn, H (2011) Why patient safety is such a tough nut to crack. *British Medical Journal*, 342: d3447.

Leonard, M, Graham, S and Bonacum, D (2004) The human factor: the critical importance of effective teamwork and communication in providing safe care. *Quality and Safety in Health Care*, 13 (suppl, 1): i85–90.

Levinson, W, Kao, A, Kuby, A and Thisted, RA (2005) Not all patients want to participate in decision-making: a national study of public preferences. *Journal of General International Medicine*, 20: 531–5.

Lilford, R, Mohammed, M, Braunholtz, D and Hofer, TP (2003) The measurement of active errors: methodological issues. *Quality and Safety in Health Care*, 12 (Suppl.II): ii8–12.

Longtin, Y, Sax, H, Leape, LL, Sheridan, SE, Donaldson, L and Pittet, D (2010) Patient participation: current knowledge and applicability to patient safety. *Mayo Clinic Proceedings*, 85: 53–62.

Lowe, CJ, Raynor, DK, Purvis, J, Farrin, A and Hudson, J (2000) Effects of a medicine review and education programme for older people in general practice. *British Journal of Pharmacology*, 50: 172–5.

Lundin, SC (2008) *Cats – The Nine Lives of Innovation*. New York: McGraw-Hill.

Lundin, SC, Christensen, J and Paul, H (2011) *Fish! A remarkable way to boost morale and improve results*. London: Hodder and Stoughton.

Lyons, M (2007) Should patients have a role in improving patient safety? A safety engineering view. *Quality and Safety in Health Care*, 16: 140–2.

McCullough, M (2011) An ethicist's journey as a patient: are we sliding down the slippery slope to sloppy healthcare? *BMJ Quality and Safety*, 20: 983–5.

McGrath, BM and Tempier, RP (2003) Implementing quality management in psychiatry: from theory to practice – shifting focus from process to outcome. *Canadian Journal of Psychiatry*, 48: 467–74.

McKimm, J and Forrest, K (eds) (2011) *Professional Practice for Foundation Doctors*. Exeter: Learning Matters.

Maher, L, Plsek, P, Garrett, S and Bevan, H (2010) *Thinking Differently*. Coventry: NHS Institute for Innovation and Improvement.

Medicines and Healthcare products Regulatory Agency (2011a) *Devices in Practice*. www.mhra.gov.uk/Publications/Safetyguidance/ Otherdevicesafetyguidance/CON007423.

Medicines and Healthcare products Regulatory Agency (2011b) *Report on Devices Adverse Incidents in 2010*. www.mhra.gov.uk/Publications/Safetyguidance/ DeviceBulletins/CON111657.

Mohr, JJ, Abelson, H and Barack, P (2002) Creating effective leadership for improving patient safety. *Quality Management in Health Care*, 11(1): 69–78.

Naessens, JM, Campbell, CR, Huddleston, JM, Berg, BP, Lefante, JJ, Williams, AR and Culbertson, RA (2009) A comparison of hospital adverse events identified by three widely used detection methods. *International Journal of Quality Health Care*, 21: 301–7.

National Audit Office (2005) *A Safer Place for Patients: Learning to improve patient safety*.

National Institute for Health and Clinical Excellence (2006) Management of Hypertension in Adults in Primary Care. Clinical Guideline 34. The National Collaborating Centre for Chronic Conditions and the British Hypertension Society. Access at www.nice.org.uk/nicemedia/pdf/cg034quickrefguide.pdf

National Patient Safety Agency (2004) *Seven Steps to Patient Safety*. July, p. 17.

National Patient Safety Agency (2007) *Observatory Report: Slips, Trips and Falls in Hospital*. Access at www.nrls.npsa.nhs.uk/resources/?entryid45=59821

National Patient Safety Agency (2008) *Patient Safety Incident Reports in the NHS: National reporting and learning system data summary*. Issue 9: August 2008, England. www.nrls.npsa.nhs.uk/resources/collections/quarterly-data-summaries/.

National Patient Safety Agency (2009) *NPSA Safety Alert, WHO Surgical Safety Checklist*. Central alert system reference NPSA/2009/PSA003. Accessed at www.nrls.npsa.nhs.uk/resources/?EntryId45=59860/ on 25 May 2012.

National Patient Safety Agency (2010) *Design for Patient Safety. User testing in the development of medical devices.* www.nrls.npsa.nhs.uk/design.

National Patient Safety Agency (2011) *Safer Spinal (Intrathecal), Epidural and Regional Devices. Part A: update.* www.nrls.npsa.nhs.uk/resources/?EntryId45=94529.

NHS Chief Executive (2011) *Innovation Review – Call for evidence and ideas.* London: Department of Health.

Nielsen, J (1994) *Usability Engineering*. Boston: AP Professional.

Norman, DA and Draper, SW (eds) (1986) *User Centered System Design: New perspectives on human–computer interaction.* Hillsdale, NJ: Erlbaum.

O'Flynn, N and Britten, N (2006) Does the achievement of medical identity limit the ability of primary care practitioners to be patient-centred? A qualitative study. *Patient Education and Counseling*, 1: 49–56.

Patient Safety First (2008) www.patientsafetyfirst.nhs.uk/ashx/Asset.ashx?path=/Patient%20Safety%20First%20-%20the%20campaign%20review.pdf, accessed 9 October 2011.

Perla, RJ, Provost, LP and Murray, SK (2011) The run chart: a simple analytical tool for learning from variation in healthcare processes. *BMJ Quality and Safety in Health Care*, 20: 46–51.

Perrow, C (1984) *Normal Accidents: Living with high-risk technologies, with a new afterword and a postscript on the y2k problem*. Princeton, NJ: Princeton University Press.

Plamping, D, Gordon, P and Pratt, J (2009) *Innovation and Public Services: Insights from evolution.* Leeds: University of Leeds, Centre for Innovation and Health Management.

Plsek, E (1997) *Creativity, Innovation and Quality.* Milwaukee: ASQ Quality Press.

Porter, RE and Samovar, LA (1991) Basic principles of intercultural communication, in Samovar, LA and Porter, RE (eds) *Intercultural Communication: A reader*, 6th edition. Belmont, CA: Wadsworth.

Pronovost, PJ and Colantuoni, E (2009) Measuring preventable harm: helping science keep pace with policy. *Journal of the American Medical Association*, 25(301): 1273–5.

Pronovost, P, Holzmueller, CG, Needham, DM, Sexton, JB, Miller, M, Berenholtz, S, Wu, AW *et al.* (2006) How will we know patients are safer? An organization-wide approach to measuring and improving safety. *Critical Care Medicine*, 34(7): 1988–95.

Pronovost, PJ, Goeschel, CA, Marsteller, JA, Sexton, JB, Pham, JC and Berenholtz, SM (2009) Framework for patient safety research and improvement. *Circulation*, 119: 330–7.

Ranji, SR and Shojania, KG (2008) Implementing patient safety interventions in your hospital: what to try and what to avoid. *Medical Clinics of North America*, 92: 275–93.

Reader, T, Flin, R and Cuthbertson, B (2007) Communication skills and error in the intensive care unit. *Current Opinions in Critical Care*, 13(6): 732–6.

Reason, J (1990) *Human Error*. New York: Cambridge University Press.

Reason, JT (1997) *Managing the Risks of Organisational Accidents*. Aldershot: Ashgate.

Reason, J (2000) Human error: models and management. *British Medical Journal*, 320(7237): 768.

Rogers, Y, Sharp, H and Preece, J (2011) *Interaction Design: Beyond human–computer interaction*. Hoboken, NJ: Wiley.

Runciman, WB, Roughead, EE, Semple, SJ and Adams, RJ (2003) Adverse drug events and medication errors in Australia. *International Journal of Quality in Health Care*, 15(Suppl. 1): i49–59.

Sari, AB, Cracknell, A and Sheldon, TA (2008) Incidence, preventability and consequences of adverse events in older people: results of a retrospective case-note review. *Age and Ageing* 37: 265–9.

Sawka, AM, Straus, S, Gafni, A, Meiyappan, S, O'Brien, MA, Brierley, JD, Tsang, RW *et al.* (2011) A usability study of a computerized decision aid to help patients with early stage papillary thyroid carcinoma in decision-making on adjuvant radioactive iodine treatment. *Patient Education and Counseling*, 84 (2): e24–7.

Scally, G and Donaldson, LJ (1998) Clinical governance and the drive for quality improvement in the new NHS in England. *British Medical Journal*, 317: 61–5.

Schein, E (1992) *Organisational Culture and Leadership*, 2nd edition. San Francisco: Jossey-Bass.

Schwappach, DLB (2010) Engaging patients as vigilant partners in safety: a systematic review. *Medical Care Research and Review*, 67: 119–48.

Schwappach, DLB and Wernli, M (2010) Chemotherapy patients' perceptions of drug administration safety. *Journal of Clinical Oncology*, 28: 2896–901.

Scott, SD, Hirschinger, LE, Cox, KR, McCoig, M, Brandt, J and Hall, LW (2009) The natural history of recovery for the healthcare provider 'second victim' after adverse patient events. *Quality and Safety in Healthcare*, 18: 325–30.

Scott, T, Mannion, R, Davies, H and Marshall, M (2003) The quantitative measurement of organisational culture in health care: a review of the available instruments. *Health Services Research*, 38(3): 923–45.

Slater, B, Lawton, R, Armitage, G, Bibby, J and Wright, J (2012) Training and action for patient safety: embedding interprofessional education for patient safety within an improvement methodology. *Journal of Continuing Education in the Health Professions*, 32(2): 80–9.

Stone, A, Slade, R, Fuller, C, Charlett, A, Cookson, B, Teare, L, Jeanes, A *et al.* (2007) Early communication: does a national campaign to improve hand hygiene in the NHS work? Initial English and Welsh experience from the NOSEC study (National Observational Study to Evaluate the Clean Your Hands Campaign). *Journal of Hospital Infection*, 66(3): 293–6.

Stoves, J, Connolly, J, Cheung, CK, Grange, A, Rhodes, P, O'Donoghue, D and Wright, J (2010) Electronic consultation as an alternative to hospital referral for patients with chronic kidney disease: a novel application for networked electronic health records to improve accessibility and efficiency of healthcare. *Quality and Safety in Health Care*, 19: e54.

Sutcliffe, K, Lewton, E and Rosenthal, M (2004) Communication failures: an insidious contributor to medical mishaps. *Academic Medicine*, 79(2): 186–94.

Sweet, SJ and Norman, IJ (1995) The nurse–doctor relationship: a selective literature review. *Journal of Advanced Nursing*, 22(1): 165–70,

Taxis, K and Barber, N (2003) Ethnographic study of incidence and severity of intravenous drug errors. *British Medical Journal*, 326: 684–7.

Thimbleby, H and Cairns, P (2010) Reducing number entry errors: solving a widespread, serious problem. *Journal of the Royal Society Interface*, 7: 1429–39.

Thomas, EJ and Petersen, LA (2003) Measuring errors and adverse events in health care. *Journal of General Internal Medicine*, 18(1): 61–7.

Toft, B (2001) *External Inquiry into the Adverse Incident that Occurred at Queen's Medical Centre, Nottingham, 4th January 2001*. Department of Health, UK. www.dh.gov.uk/en/Publicationsandstatistics/Publications/PublicationsPolicyAndGuidance/DH_4010064.

Van den Bemt, PMLA, Egberts, ACG, Lenderink, AW, Verzijl, JM, Simons, KA, Van der Pol, WS and Leufkens, HG (1999) Adverse drug events in hospitalized patients: a comparison of doctors, nurses and patients as sources of reports. *Pharmacoepidemiology and Prescription*, 55: 155–8.

Villette, M (2011) For want of a four-cent pull chain. *BMJ Quality Safety*, 20: 986–90.

Vincent, C (2010) *Patient Safety*. Chichester: Wiley-Blackwell/BMJ Books.

Vincent, C and Coulter, A (2002) Patient safety: what about the patient? *Quality and Safety in Health Care*, 11: 76–80.

Wald, H, and Shojania, KG (2003) *Incident Reporting. Building foundations, reducing risk agency for healthcare research and quality*. Rockville, MD: Agency for Healthcare Research and Quality.

Walker, S (2004) Settling medical negligence disputes: now and in the future. Conference Paper at Making Health Care Safer 22 October, Royal College of Physicians of London.

Ward, JK and Armitage, G (2012) Can patients report patient safety incidents in a hospital setting? *BMJ Quality and Safety*: 1–5. Available at http://qualitysafety. bmj.com/content/early/2012/05/04/bmjqs-2011-000213.full

Ward, JR and Clarkson, PJ (2007) Human factors engineering and the design of medical devices, in Carayon, P (ed.) *Handbook of Human Factors and Ergonomics in Health Care and Patient Safety*. Mahwah, NJ: Lawrence Erlbaum.

Ward, JK, McEachan, RRC, Lawton, R, Armitage, G, Watt, I and Wright, J (2011) Patient involvement in patient safety: protocol for developing an intervention using patient reports of organisational safety and patient incident reporting. *BMC Health Services Research*, 11: 130.

Waterman, AD, Gallagher, TH, Garbutt, J, Waterman, BM, Fraser, V and Burroughs, TE (2006) Hospitalized patients' attitudes about and participation in error prevention. *Journal of General International Medicine*, 21: 367–70.

Waterworth, S and Luker, KA (1990) Reluctant collaborators: do patients want to be involved in decisions concerning care? *Journal of Advanced Nursing*, 15: 971–6.

Weingart, SN, Pagovich, O, Sands, DZ, Li, JM, Aronson, MD, Davis, RB and Bates, DW (2005) What can hospitalized patients tell us about adverse events? Learning from patient-reported incidents. *Journal of General Internatinal Medicine*, 20: 830–6.

Weingart, SN, Price, J, Duncombe, D, Connor, M, Sommer, K, Conley, KA, Bierer, BE *et al*. (2007) Patient-reported safety and quality of care in outpatient oncology. *Joint Commission Journal on Quality Patient Safety*, 33: 83–93.

Weissman, JS, Schneider, EC, Weingart, SN, Epstein, AM, David-Kasdan, J, Feibelmann, S, Annas, CL *et al*. (2008) Comparing patient-reported hospital adverse events with medical record review: do patients know something that hospitals do not? *Annals of Internal Medicine*, 149: 100–8.

Willems, S, De Maesschalck, S, Deveugele, M, Derese, A and De Maeseneer, J (2005) Socio-economic status of the patient and doctor–patient communication: does it make a difference? *Patient Education and Counseling,* 56: 139–46.

Winterbottom, AE, Jha, V, Melville, C, Corrado, O, Symons, J, Torgerson, D, Watt, I *et al.* (2010) A randomised controlled trial of patient led training in medical education: protocol. *BMC Medical Education,* 10: 90.

Wong, BM, Etchells, EE, Kuper, A, Levinson, W and Shojania, KG (2010) Teaching quality improvement and patient safety to trainees: a systematic review. *Academic Medicine,* 85(9): 1425–39.

Woods, DD and Cook, RI (2002) Nine steps to move forward from error. *Cognitive Technology and Work,* 4(2): 137–44.

World Health Organization (2009) *Patient Safety Curriculum Guide for Medical Schools.* Geneva: WHO.

World Health Organization (2011) *Patient Safety Curriculum Guide: Multiprofessional education.* Geneva: WHO.

Wu, AW (2000) Medical error: the second victim. *British Medical Journal,* 320 (7237): 726.

Zhang, J, Johnson, TR, Patel, VL, Paige, DL and Kubose, T (2003) Using usability heuristics to evaluate patient safety of medical devices. *Journal of Biomedical Informatics,* 36(1–2): 23–30.

Index